Field and Ambulatory Medicine

Editor

ADOLF K. MAAS III

VETERINARY CLINICS
OF NORTH AMERICA:
EXOTIC ANIMAL PRACTICE

www.vetexotic.theclinics.com

Consulting Editor
JÖRG MAYER

September 2018 • Volume 21 • Number 3

ELSEVIER

1600 John F. Kennedy Boulevard ● Suite 1800 ● Philadelphia, Pennsylvania, 19103-2899
http://www.vetexotic.theclinics.com

VETERINARY CLINICS OF NORTH AMERICA: EXOTIC ANIMAL PRACTICE Volume 21, Number 3
September 2018 ISSN 1094-9194, ISBN-13: 978-0-323-61416-0

Editor: Colleen Dietzler
Developmental Editor: Meredith Madeira

Veterinary Clinics of North America: Exotic Animal Practice (ISSN 1094-9194) is published in January, May, and September by Elsevier, Inc., 360 Park Avenue South, New York, NY 10010-1710. Subscription prices are $276.00 per year for US individuals, $492.00 per year for US institutions, $100.00 per year for US students and residents, $324.00 per year for Canadian individuals, $593.00 per year for Canadian institutions, $347.00 per year for international individuals, $593.00 per year for international institutions and $165.00 per year for Canadian and foreign students/ residents. To receive student/resident rate, orders must be accompanied by name of affiliated institution, date of term, and the *signature* of program/residency coordinator on institution letterhead. Orders will be billed at individual rate until proof of status is received. Foreign air speed delivery is included in all *Clinics* subscription prices. All prices are subject to change without notice. **POSTMASTER:** Send address changes to *Veterinary Clinics of North America: Exotic Animal Practice*, Elsevier Health Sciences Division, Subscription Customer Service, 3251 Riverport Lane, Maryland Heights, MO 63043. **Customer Service: Telephone: 1-800-654-2452** (U.S. and Canada); **1-314-447-8871** (outside U.S. and Canada). **Fax: 1-314-447-8029. E-mail: journalscustomerservice-usa@elsevier.com (for print support); journalsonlinesupport-usa@elsevier.com (for online support).**

Reprints. For copies of 100 or more of articles in this publication, please contact the Commercial Reprints Department, Elsevier Inc., 360 Park Avenue South, New York, New York 10010-1710. Tel.: 212-633-3874; Fax: 212-633-3820; E-mail: reprints@elsevier.com.

Veterinary Clinics of North America: Exotic Animal Practice is covered in *MEDLINE/PubMed (Index Medicus).*

Contributors

CONSULTING EDITOR

JÖRG MAYER, Dr med vet, Msc
Diplomate, American Board of Veterinary Practitioners (Exotic Companion Mammals); Diplomate, European College of Zoological Medicine (Small Mammals); Diplomate, American College of Zoological Medicine; Associate Professor of Zoological Medicine, Department of Small Animal Medicine and Surgery, University of Georgia College of Veterinary Medicine, Athens, Georgia

EDITOR

ADOLF K. MAAS III, DVM, CertAqVet
Diplomate, American Board of Veterinary Practitioners (Reptile and Amphibian Medicine and Surgery); Director of Veterinary Medicine and Nutrition, Toledo Zoo, Toledo, Ohio; ZooVet Consulting, PLLC, Bothell, Washington

AUTHORS

JAMES E. BOGAN Jr, DVM, CertAqV
Diplomate, American Board of Veterinary Practitioners (Canine and Feline Practice); Diplomate, American Board of Veterinary Practitioners (Reptile and Amphibian Practice); Owner, The Critter Fixer of Central Florida, Oviedo, Florida

RICHARD GREGORY BURKETT, DVM
Diplomate, American Board of Veterinary Practitioners (Avian Practice); Owner and Operator, The Bird Hospital: Avian Veterinary Services, The Birdie Boutique, Inc, Durham, North Carolina

SATHYA K. CHINNADURAI, DVM, MS
Diplomate, American College of Zoological Medicine; Diplomate, American College of Veterinary Anesthesia and Analgesia; Senior Staff Veterinarian, Brookfield Zoo, Chicago Zoological Society, Brookfield, Illinois; Adjunct Clinical Assistant Professor, University of Illinois College of Veterinary Medicine, Urbana, Illinois

TODD DRIGGERS, DVM
Avian and Exotic Animal Clinic of Arizona, Mesa, Arizona

RICHARD S. FUNK, MA, DVM
Adjunct Professor of Veterinary Clinical Sciences, College of Veterinary Medicine, Midwestern University, Glendale, Arizona; Richard Funk Veterinary Services LLC, Mesa, Arizona

DAVID HANNON, DVM
Diplomate, American Board of Veterinary Practitioners (Avian); Avian and Exotic Animal Veterinary Services, PetVax Complete Care Centers, Memphis, Tennessee

KENDAL E. HARR, DVM, MS
Diplomate, American College of Veterinary Pathologists; URIKA, LLC, Mukilteo, Washington

SUSAN HORTON, DVM
Chief of Staff, Chicago Exotics Animal Hospital, Skokie, Illinois

ADOLF K. MAAS III, DVM, CertAqVet
Diplomate, American Board of Veterinary Practitioners (Reptile and Amphibian Medicine and Surgery); Director of Veterinary Medicine and Nutrition, Toledo Zoo, Toledo, Ohio; ZooVet Consulting, PLLC, Bothell, Washington

ERICA MEDE, CVT
Head Certified Veterinary Technician, Exotic, Zoo, and Wildlife, Chicago Exotics Animal Hospital, Skokie, Illinois; President, Friends of Scales Reptile Rescue, Wheeling, Illinois

JANE E. MEIER, DVM
Bonita, California

JESSIE SANDERS, DVM, CertAqV
Aquatic Veterinary Services, Watsonville, California

DANIELLE STRAHL-HELDRETH, MS, DVM
Resident in Anesthesiology, University of Illinois College of Veterinary Medicine, Veterinary Teaching Hospital, Urbana, Illinois

BRADLEY J. WAFFA, MSPH, DVM
Gentle Care Animal Hospital, Raleigh, North Carolina

Contents

> Ambulatory veterinary practice is anything but a new concept; although it was not a significant portion of companion animal medicine for the last 5 decades, it has been and continues to be the mainstay of large animal practice. As exotic animal medicine has been one of the fastest growing segments of veterinary medicine, mobile and on-site care for these nontraditional species (both pets and collection based) is a rapidly growing segment of on-demand veterinary care. With good planning, organization, and equipment, ambulatory medical services can provide as good care as what can be practiced in any stationary practice.

> The diversity of species and habitats encountered in nontraditional veterinary practice lends itself to a passionate veterinarian with a wide-ranging set of surgical, medical, and husbandry skills. At every appointment, exotic animal veterinarians perform 2 examinations (patient and environment). The animal and environmental examinations often identify relationships that lend themselves to appropriate medical care and therapies. This article gives practical knowledge and experience to the veterinary professional for the purpose of building an ambulatory service to enhance the success of or to create a stationary practice.

> The ambulatory exotic animal practice provides a unique paradigm within veterinary medicine, one with new challenges and great rewards and benefits. In today's world, however, every practitioner needs to be cognizant of the legal issues and liabilities that may befall them and plan accordingly. Ambulatory nontraditional species practice has additional legal risks and concerns. This article provides information so that the veterinarian can make educated decisions while reducing their liability.

> Veterinary technicians are continuously evolving with changes in veterinary medicine specialties. Traditionally, ambulatory medicine has focused on large farm animal medicine. In today's world, technicians are finding themselves on house calls and in ambulatory practices that focus on exotic and

zoologic species. In ambulatory medicine, technicians assist during field surgery work, on-site diagnostics, and in other various roles. The conditions often are not ideal and require attention to detail to avoid mistakes in record keeping, inventory, and unnecessary risk.

Results may be changed with suboptimal sample collection and transport, which then result in incorrect diagnoses. Quality management of samples must start in the patient, extend through sampling itself, include appropriate short transport, and then be correctly accessioned at the referral laboratory or in-house station to ensure accurate diagnosis of disease. A quality assurance plan at the laboratory chosen is mandatory under American Society for Veterinary Clinical Pathology guidelines.

With the growing popularity in the ownership of nontraditional species, there is a growing need for veterinarians to be able to provide out-of-clinic health assessments on privately owned exotic species. Ambulatory anesthesia is often required for diagnostic and surgical procedures in remote or nonhospital settings. Anesthesia for diagnostic procedures is commonly used to ensure the safety of personnel and exotic veterinary patients, particularly when there is an inability to transport the animal to the clinic. The challenges of exotic animal anesthesia are further compounded by the logistical challenges of performing anesthesia outside of the hospital setting.

Ambulatory aquatic veterinary medicine allows examination of a patient's environment and identification of potentially sick animals. Common clients to use ambulatory service are owners of large koi and aquaculture facilities, but any aquatic animal owner could benefit from on-site services. This practice limits stress from handling and transporting large or critically sick or injured aquatic animals. Additional skills must be practiced to attain proficiency in capturing potential patients. Most diagnostics are available to practitioners in an ambulatory setting, and follow-up care must be thoroughly discussed with clients.

Herpetology specialists may find a rewarding model in production medicine, where patients are evaluated on a population basis in an ambulatory setting. Ambulatory medicine combines clinical advantages, such as being able to evaluate patients and their living conditions in situ, with the benefits of building close client relationships and tethering the growth of the business with that of an increasingly popular niche industry. Ambulatory medicine does present some logistical challenges when working with reptiles and amphibians, but they represent surmountable growing pains for the veterinarian committed to growing alongside the ever-evolving practice of reptile and amphibian medicine and surgery.

> An avian ambulatory practice is a veterinary practice that can be started with a small investment and has low overhead and operating expenses. It is an opportunity for veterinarians who want to open their own practice. This type of practice has advantages and disadvantages. Practitioners can set their own hours and be their own boss. They are better able accommodate clients by making it more convenient for them to schedule appointments. Practitioners can take advantage of home visits to correct environmental issues. Disadvantages center on practitioners being the sole source of income and how that affects their lives outside the practice.

> An exotic companion animal ambulatory practice has unique challenges, advantages, and disadvantages. Not all veterinarians are suited to this type of practice, but it can be exceptionally rewarding. It can also be exceptionally frustrating. Ambulatory practice offers veterinary services to those clients who for a variety of reasons do not or cannot take their exotic companion animal, potbellied pig, or llama to a veterinary practice. Being able to observe husbandry and feeding practices and an animal's environment, the mobile veterinarian gets a more well-rounded picture of the patient.

> This article reviews the necessary process an exotic veterinarian needs to understand when considering being an attending veterinarian for a United States Department of Agriculture–regulated facility.

> Owing to myriad species and their variety of needs, ambulatory zoologic practice can carry many challenges. The practitioner must be appropriately prepared, with the necessary equipment, medications, and supplies, which should either accompany the veterinarian or be available at the site where the work is performed. It is imperative that the veterinarian has proper knowledge of the care and feeding of these animals and knows and understands the legalities of owning and working with them. The ambulatory zoo veterinarian must be able to address the medical and surgical needs of these animals in a field or other nonconventional setting.

While practicing exotic animal medicine as an ambulatory practitioner, veterinarians need to be prepared for the inevitable emergency call. Emergencies in exotic animal medicine come in all shapes and sizes, and the veterinarian must be prepared for a variety of situations. With proper training, equipment, and managing client expectations, an ambulatory exotics animal practitioner can successfully address emergencies. This article provides a brief overview of managing emergency cases in an ambulatory exotics animal practice.

VETERINARY CLINICS OF NORTH AMERICA: EXOTIC ANIMAL PRACTICE

FORTHCOMING ISSUES

January 2019
Medical and Surgical Management of Ocular Surface Disease in Exotic Animals
Sarah Louise Czerwinski, *Editor*

May 2019
Orthopedics
Mikel Sabater González and Daniel Calvo Carrasco, *Editors*

September 2019
Technological Advances in Exotic Pet Practice
Minh Huynh, *Editor*

RECENT ISSUES

May 2018
Therapeutics
Yvonne R.A. van Zeeland, *Editor*

January 2018
Exotic Animal Neurology
Susan E. Orosz, *Editor*

September 2017
Evidence-based Clinical Practice in Exotic Animal Medicine
Nicola DiGirolamo and Alexandra L. Winter, *Editors*

ISSUE OF RELATED INTEREST

Veterinary Clinics: Exotic Animal Practice
May 2016, (Vol. 19, No. 2)
Emergency and Critical Care
Margaret Fordham, Brian K. Roberts, *Editors*
Available at: http://www.vetexotic.theclinics.com

THE CLINICS ARE NOW AVAILABLE ONLINE!
Access your subscription at:
www.theclinics.com

Preface

It Feels Good to Be On the Road Again

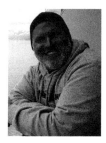

Adolf K. Maas III, DVM, CertAqVet, DABVP
(Reptile and Amphibian Medicine and Surgery)
Editor

When I started my first exotic animal ambulatory practice, a colleague told me that he thought it was a bad idea. He told me that a mobile practice for anything but large animals was an archaic means of treating patients. He felt that the only reason to do it for cows and horses was that there was no efficient way to transport them to a facility. His opinion was that to practice in anything other than a "brick-and-mortar" office limited the quality and level of medicine that could be practiced on dogs and cats, let alone on nontraditional species. The discussion ended on the note that I would soon give up, as there was no way that I could make a living, and that I would be quickly returning to the first hospital that would hire me.

A bit over a year later, we crossed paths again. I was driving the "practice vehicle," so it happened that he got a first-hand view of how it was equipped: There was a portable anesthesia machine, surgical equipment, blood chemistry analyzer, ultrasound unit, portable exam table, endoscopy, and much more, all organized in the back of my '97 Jeep Cherokee. My schedule was full, and I kept all my records on a laptop computer. Ironically, he admitted my rig was better outfitted than his "brick-and-mortar" clinic, and I do not recall him ever talking about the futility of ambulatory veterinary practice again.

I do, however, recall that this practice was a series of trial and errors. I reached out to as many compatriots as I could, but exotic animal practice was still a developing focus. There were even fewer mobile practitioners. I tried to learn from the resources that were available, but there were only so many pearls of wisdom from dairy medicine that could be carried over to high-quality exotic animal medicine. In short, the resources necessary to be able to build this type of novel practice with any skill were simply not available.

In this issue of *Veterinary Clinics of North America: Exotic Animal Practice*, the goal is to provide practitioners with the resources that will help them build and develop a high-quality exotic animal ambulatory practice. Here, we explore many of the key aspects of

https://doi.org/10.1016/j.cvex.2018.05.014
1094-9194/18/© 2018 Published by Elsevier Inc.

exotic animal mobile medicine, starting with a perspective of melding an ambulatory service into an established stationary practice. Following this are articles that review the role of veterinary technicians and how these essential members of a veterinary team can improve the quality and efficiency of practice, followed by an excellent summary of ambulatory sample collection and transport, which details how to produce the highest-quality diagnostic results. The special topic of anesthesia and how it should be applied to mobile practice is also presented to cover this complex area of ambulatory medicine. The primary facets of exotic animal practice, broken into aquatic, herpetologic, avian, and exotic companion mammal species, with discussions of the equipment and techniques needed to provide quality care needed on a mobile basis, are presented in subsequent sections. These topics are complemented by an article that looks at ambulatory zoologic medicine practice and the challenges created by these unique animals as well as by a review of a mobile exotic animal practitioner in USDA inspections and regulations, and, finally, by an overview of ambulatory practice emergency medicine, to provide the practitioner with as complete of a picture as possible.

As a fellow practitioner, I look forward to the advice and experience these authors bring to this issue, and I expect that I will learn as much as everyone else who reads these pages. I am genuinely grateful for the commitment each author has demonstrated by sharing their knowledge in order to help future veterinarians provide the best care for their patients.

I would be truly remiss to forget all the others that have played a critical part in the success of this issue. The editorial staff at Elsevier has provided the essential assistance and support to make this a worthy issue and assisted me through the process of serving as a guest editor. I also have my son, Will, to thank as he has been a great motivator to seek knowledge and excellence and to do the right thing. Most of all, I thank my wife, Kelli, who has always been my muse and inspiration, and who is forever in support of all the crazy things I do.

Adolf K. Maas III, DVM, CertAqVet, DABVP
(Reptile and Amphibian Medicine and Surgery)
Toledo Zoo
2 Hippo Drive
Toledo, Ohio 43614, USA

ZooVet Consulting, PLLC
PO Box 1007
Bothell, WA 98041, USA

E-mail address:
drmaas@zoovet.us

Ambulatory Exotic and Nontraditional Species Medicine

Adolf K. Maas III, DVM, CertAqVet, DABVP (Reptile and Amphibian Medicine and Surgery)[a,b,*]

KEYWORDS

- Ambulatory • Exotics • History • Medicine

KEY POINTS

- Veterinary medicine started with ambulatory medicine.
- Ambulatory medicine is one of the fastest growing aspects of veterinary medicine.
- Ambulatory exotic animal medicine has an essential role in veterinary medicine.
- An ambulatory practice can provide as good of, if not better, quality of medicine as a brick and mortar practice to nontraditional species patients.

Ambulatory medicine was the foundation of veterinary practice, as the first veterinarians were purely mobile, taking their materials and skills to the patients and owners. This practice was generated out of need, as the first clients were that of farmers and horsemen who needed care for their herds and flock. In an effort to maintain their livelihood and herds, it was far more feasible to bring the doctor to the patients.[1] Even the term *veterinarian* comes from the Latin *veterinarius* defined as "pertaining to the beast of burden."

James Alfred Wright, also known as James Herriott,[2] both romanticized as well as practiced ambulatory medicine at the height of its extent. In his memoirs, he described the transition of small animal practice from primarily farm and house calls to the expansion of the brick and mortar practice while facilitating the separation of small animal from large animal practice.[2]

Despite human medicine continuing the practice of house calls for patients, veterinary house call medicine declined much sooner, as brick and mortar was chosen for ease and simplicity. The concept of taking the pet to the vet rather than the vet to the pet was preferred for many reasons, not the least of which was to increase efficiency; provide support staff; and, because much of early small animal veterinary

Disclosure: The author has nothing to disclose.
[a] Toledo Zoo, 2 Hippo Drive, Toledo, Ohio 43614, USA; [b] ZooVet Consulting, PLLC, PO Box 1007, Bothell, WA 98041, USA
* ZooVet Consulting, PLLC, PO Box 1007, Bothell, WA 98041.
E-mail address: DrMaas@zoovet.us

care was surgical, to provide a dedicated and controlled environment for safe and effective procedures.

Since then, to say that veterinary medicine has changed is nothing but an understatement. Veterinary doctors now have so much more available to their patients than providing empirical care based on presentation and symptoms (not to undervalue these aspects, in any way) and basic surgical care as the extent of the therapy that could be provided. As clinicians, there is the offering of extensive biochemical and hematologic testing; assessments of hormone levels; genetic and cytochemical marker testing for countless diseases; imaging techniques with the ability to identify internal structures and pathologies as, if not more, detailed than with open approaches; therapies that pioneer treatments in human medicine; and surgical techniques rivaling that of any medical center. And all of this is readily available to any clinician (**Fig. 1**).

With this, there has been the return to ambulatory medicine over the last couple of decades. The North American Veterinary Conference group has listed this as one of the fastest growing segments of veterinary medicine,[3] with demand often outstripping supply. Mobile hospitals are readily available and affordable, with both initial as well as long-term costs much lower than that of traditional clinics. Their growth has been so rapid that many states have been adding specific rules and requirements to their veterinary board regulations so that the care and services provided are ensured to meet the same practice standards of care as any other veterinarian. A recent visit to 2 major veterinary medical conferences by the author identified at least 6 distinct companies/franchises recruiting veterinarians to staff mobile veterinary practices covering both the Western and Eastern United States, with rapidly growing clienteles and practices.[4] In fact, many of these mobile hospitals are better equipped than their stationary counterparts; there are those that already offer services beyond the typical routine practice.[5]

Thus, not with a purr but with a roar has been the return of ambulatory medicine to small animal practice.

Ambulatory nontraditional species medicine is, however, a relatively new development within the aspect of veterinary medicine. This new development is primarily because exotic animal medicine (other than zoo animal medicine) is also a relatively new addition to veterinary practice that has experienced massive growth in the last 30 years. Starting in the 1950s and 1960s was the serious development of zoo animal medicine[6] with the establishment of the American Association of Zoologic

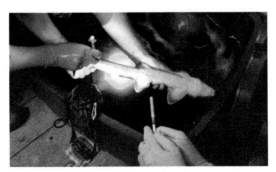

Fig. 1. All manners of patients will be encountered with ambulatory exotic animal practice. Here, blood is being collected from a shark for analysis. (*Courtesy of* Adolf K. Maas III, DVM, Bothell, WA.)

Veterinarians as both a resource and a forum to share ideas and experiences, followed by the development of the first text on zoo animal medicine and the formation of zoo medicine specialist qualifications. This development expanded the knowledge base of the care of these unique animals; as nontraditional species began to become more popular in private collections and households in the 1980s, the recognition that these animals were also not simply disposable and experienced not only unique conditions and pathologies but they also required unique care and treatment fomented the development of several collectives of veterinarians who wanted to study and develop evidence-based medicine for their patients (**Fig. 2**).

The 1990s and early 2000s saw the most dramatic growth of groups dedicated to the medicine of these (often nondomesticated) species. The Association of Avian Veterinarians and the Association of Reptile and Amphibian Veterinarians were well established and growing. From growing need and knowledge, the Association of the Exotic Mammal Veterinarians was formed. Many seminal editions of

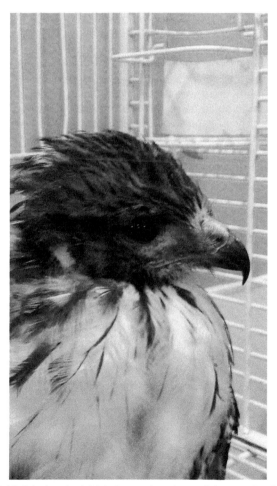

Fig. 2. A falconer's bird during the initial observation phase of the examination, resting fluffed and comfortably but obviously not well. (*Courtesy of* Adolf K. Maas III, DVM, Bothell, WA.)

textbooks discussing diseases and treatments of these groups of animals were published, demonstrating that diagnosis and therapy no longer had to be empirical and speculative.[7–9] With these texts, veterinary groups, and the knowledge that they encouraged and shared, the practice of exotic animal/nontraditional species formally took shape and grew. Partnerships with the American Board of Veterinary Practitioners developed guidelines for minimum specialist knowledge bases to create taxa-specific specialist certification within each of these groups (**Fig. 3**).

As the practice of exotic animal medicine grew, so grew the practitioners that reached out into this branch. Many of them practiced their arts as part of their small animal practice, branching out as the ultimate in mixed-animal practice, whereas a few brave souls opened practices that were dedicated to the exclusive care of reptiles, birds, and exotic mammals. As one might assume, however, these practices were few and far between and often had initial narrow budgets, as their clients were less populous and it was often challenging to charge appropriate rates for an animal often considered more easily replaced.

One option that was reincarnated, because of both a smaller initial as well as ongoing financial investment, was to return to ambulatory services. There was no real estate cost, as the family sports utility vehicle (SUV), minivan, or station wagon could readily be double purposed as a mobile office, reducing costs of business easily 20%. Staff was inexistent to minimal, as the receptionist and front desk were replaced by the cellular phone and few early mobile practitioners required full-time technical staff. There were no kennels, thus, no kennel staff or food services required. Records could be easily kept on paper; but with the growing availability and affordability of laptop computers and portable printers and power converters, this soon grew as the preferred modality requiring little to no space. Storage systems could be built or purchased to accommodate all the diagnostic, sample collection, pharmaceutical, and even surgical equipment needed; the

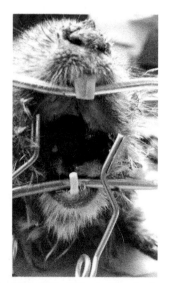

Fig. 3. An anesthetized chinchilla (*Chinchilla lanigera*) about to undergo treatment of gingival hyperplasia. Herbivore dental work is a relatively common procedure performed in the field. (*Courtesy of* Adolf K. Maas III, DVM, DABVP, Bothell, WA.)

practitioner could grow the practice (equipment, offerings, and clientele) as they wished and finances allowed. In short, for a small fraction of both the initial and continuing expense (as low as only 10%–30% of a stationary practice), skilled and confident exotic-animal veterinarians could hang their shingle and immediately provide quality service to their clients and patients.

Many early nontraditional species practitioners started their practices in this manner. By offering mobile medical services, these practitioners could overcome many of the issues faced by clients (transport of larger animals, challenging patients, collections within facilities, accessing distant or remote locations) all while being able to provide veterinary services by a doctor whose knowledge and skill set applied more specifically to the patients at hand. Through relationships with stationary (dog and cat) practices, they were able to provide expanded services that were either not offered or feasible in mobile services (radiology, ultrasonography, surgery, hospitalization, and laboratory services, depending on the setup of the particular mobile practice) (**Fig. 4**).

How these practices developed as they grew varied, however. Some of them remained mobile and continue to this day as exclusively ambulatory practitioners. These practices may be operating out of a vehicle (van/SUV/wagon) or have changed to a mobile home style unit or they have built relationships with the facilities they service and have multiple transient clinics at each of them (such as are described in the "Ambulatory Zoo Practice" article in this issue). Others have transitioned to stationary practices with active mobile services as needed. A few have established clinics to provide necessary stationary services but are still primarily ambulatory practices. Lastly, a few have taken highly successful ambulatory practices and opened comparably successful brick-and-mortar hospitals while ceasing all off-site services.

Although these are all referring to practices in the historical sense, it is easy to see how this can not only be repeated with great success but also continues to be in current events. Several studies[10–12] have found that whereas the general attitude of veterinary clients do not expect the average veterinarian to offer extended hours of operations while concurrently expecting specialists to be available later in the day as well as on weekends to accommodate work schedules and offer more conveniences, linked to higher charges of the specialists. The prospect of providing exotic animal care and services on a mobile basis is highly desirable by the average clientele, and most clients are willing to pay a premium for this additional service.

Just as there are advantages to the client to provide ambulatory services, there are also significant advantages to the practitioner as a person. Ambulatory practitioners

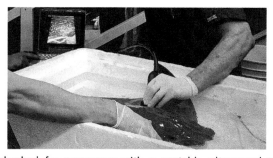

Fig. 4. A ray is checked for pregnancy with a portable ultrasound unit. This type of procedure all but requires ambulatory services because of the difficulty of transporting patients. (*Courtesy of* Adolf K. Maas III, DVM, Bothell, WA.)

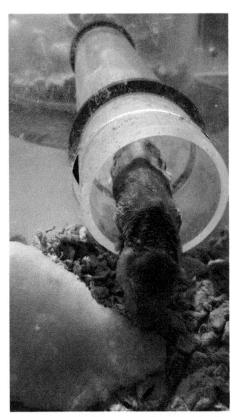

Fig. 5. Ambulatory exotic animal medicine greatly expands the opportunity to work with uncommon species. Here, a naked mole rat (*Heterocephalus glaber*) emerges from a tube in its enclosure before examination. (*Courtesy of* Adolf K. Maas III, DVM, Bothell, WA.)

have the ability to work as much or as little as they prefer and can base it on the time of year or around other commitments. Growth of the practice can be their decision, such as whether they only take prearranged visits, work only with commercial operations, manage their own emergency work, and determine the territories they want to cover. They have the autonomy to make decisions regarding equipment and staff as well as have more control over the advancement of their skills and knowledge and the species/patients that they attend to. In many ways, the work/life balance is more in their own hands. These advantages are, however, not even including the advantages provided to them as clinicians and the benefits of examining their patients in their own territory (**Fig. 5**).

Nontraditional species medicine includes all types of animals in all types of situations and, thus, allows for an immense opportunity for field clinicians to develop their practice as they wish to pursue. The ambulatory clinician can choose to focus on aquatic animal medicine, avian practice, herpetological medicine, exotic companion mammals, zoologic collections, regulatory medicine, wildlife rehabilitation or any possible mix of any or all of these groups. There are no limitations based on animal size, habitat, or any other issues that hamper practice within a stationary facility. Other things that are performed in a brick-and-mortar practice are possible, whether it be radiology or ultrasonography, behavior and internal medicine, anesthesia and surgery, oncological therapy, or any other aspect of veterinary medicine. With recent advancements in portable diagnostic laboratories, imaging, and anesthesia monitoring equipment, and the application of newer ambulatory practice designs, the standard of care can be not only met but exceeded in virtually any situation, for any patient (**Fig. 6**).

As with all areas of exotic animal practice, there are risks and concerns that should be managed before they become an issue. Zoonoses are always a factor in veterinary medicine, and the incidence and occurrence increase when working with nontraditional species and increase even more when the practitioner has the opportunity to involve him or herself with the environment that the patients live within. Some diseases, like herpes B virus, have minimal pathological processes in host nonhuman primates but are fatal to humans who are infected. Reverse zoonoses are also as much of a risk to patients, as human herpes simplex virus most commonly only causes cold sores and oral zosters in people but is a fatal infection to nonhuman primates that are inadvertently infected. There is also the risk of the veterinarian becoming the source of a disease; just as what is practiced within large animal medicine, the doctors must take additional precautions to disinfect themselves to prevent the transmission of pathogens not only from one site to another but also from a asymptomatic carrier animal to a susceptible host (**Fig. 7**).

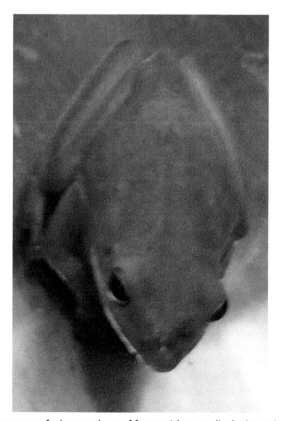

Fig. 6. This frog was one of a large colony of frogs with most displaying raised red lesions on various areas of their body. These lesions tested positive for *Mycobacterium chelonae* as well as their enclosure. The handlers required testing, with one individual requiring surgical removal of a lesion. (*Courtesy of* Adolf K. Maas III, DVM, Bothell, WA.)

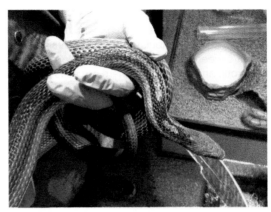

Fig. 7. Proper protective gear should be worn when examining any patient. (*Courtesy of* Adolf K. Maas III, DVM, Bothell, WA.)

Right now the cornerstone is being built for ambulatory nontraditional species medicine. As mobile services are well established for equine, small ruminant, and bovine medicine, entrepreneurial exotic animal veterinarians can draw from the wealth of experience and information that is available.[13,14] There is a growing body of information on building and managing on-site/on-demand companion animal veterinary practices, with resources readily available.[15] Simply put, the resources are there, the equipment is there, and the demand is there. All it needs is the addition of a talented, knowledgeable, independent veterinarian to catalyze the idea into a successful practice.

REFERENCES

1. Boyd CT. The lost history of American veterinary medicine: the need for preservation. J Med Libr Assoc 2011;99(1):8–14.
2. Herriott J. All creatures great and small. New York: Bantam Doubleday Dell; 1972.
3. Available at: http://navc.com/spark/list/wjGCwiuF/video/9nA0orNe/on-demand-veterinary-care. Accessed January 29, 2018.
4. VMX, 2018, and Western Veterinary Conference, 2018.
5. Available at: http://todaysveterinarypractice.navc.com/the-back-page-veterinary-viewpointsthe-house-call-veterinarian/. Accessed February 14, 2018.
6. History of the AAZV. Available at: http://www.aazv.org/?35. Accessed December 1, 2017.
7. Ritchie BW, Harrison JG, Harrison RL. Avian medicine. Lake Worth (FL): Winger's Publishing. Inc; 1994.
8. Mader DR. Reptile medicine and surgery. 1996.
9. Quesenberry KE, Carpenter JW. Ferrets, rabbits, and rodents: clinical medicine and surgery. 2004.
10. Gregório H, Santos P, Pires I, et al. Comparison of veterinary health services expectations and perceptions between oncologic pet owners, non-oncologic pet owners and veterinary staff using the SERVQUAL methodology. Vet World 2016;9(11):1275–81. https://doi.org/10.14202/vetworld.2016.1275-1281.
11. Coe JB, Adams CL, Bonnett BN. A focus group study of veterinarians' and pet owners' perceptions of the monetary aspects of veterinary care. J Am Vet Med Assoc 2007;231(10):1510–8.

12. Herron ME, Lord LK. Use of and satisfaction of pet owners with a clinical behavior service in a companion animal specialty referral practice. J Am Vet Med Assoc 2012;241(11):1463–6.
13. Ramey DW, Baus MR. Ambulatory practice. Vet Clin North Am Equine Pract 2012; 1:xi–xii.
14. Tricks M. The costs and considerations of establishing a mobile equine veterinary clinic in Wells, Somerset, UK (Doctoral dissertation). 2014.
15. Available at: https://www.aaha.org/marketconnect/company?com=American_ Association_of_Mobile_Veterinary_Practitioners. Accessed March 1, 2018.

Incorporating/Integrating Exotic Ambulatory Medicine into a Brick-and-Mortar Practice

Todd Driggers, DVM

KEYWORDS

- Exotics • Mobile • Veterinary practice • Medicine • Surgery • Avian • Reptilian
- Mammalian

KEY POINTS

- When creating an ambulatory practice, vision, core vision, goals, and related business plans need to be clearly defined.
- Both practice types have clear advantages and disadvantages.
- Successful management of an ambulatory practice can create the venue for a stationary practice and vice-versa.
- Stationary practices cannot replace the insights gained by a well-organized ambulatory practice.

INTRODUCTION

Little is found in literature about the evolution of an exotic ambulatory service into a fully functioning stationary practice or the converse of "brick-and-mortar" practices developing mobile services: experience, Internet searches, and opinions from colleagues are the start of what is likely to become a more completely reviewed topic in the future. Application of these ideas, principles, and philosophies regarding successful establishment of an ambulatory veterinary exotic practice may enable practitioners to reach individual goals outlined in their vision and mission statements. Ideally, combining both ambulatory and stationary practice types give clinicians the best opportunity to provide nontraditional species patients appropriate evidence-based care.

What constitutes an "exotic animal" is relatively unclear. By contrast, the definition of domestic animals is those selectively bred and habituated to human needs and purposes in a captive environment.[1] All veterinarians receive training in domestic animal husbandry, medicine, and surgery, primarily dogs, cats, cows, and horses. Also

Disclosure: The author has nothing to disclose.
Avian and Exotic Animal Clinic of Arizona, 1911 South Lindsay Road, Mesa, AZ 85204, USA
E-mail address: todddriggers@mac.com

Vet Clin Exot Anim 21 (2018) 539–549
https://doi.org/10.1016/j.cvex.2018.05.002
1094-9194/18/© 2018 Elsevier Inc. All rights reserved.

included are the common domestic farm animals that are considered production animals and not pets.

"Exotics," within the vernacular of veterinary medicine, are often animals that exist in the wild, but also may be domesticated. Captive breeding of wild species is often an early process of domestication, but history has shown that not all species, despite best efforts, can be domesticated. Color morphs, patterns, size differences, tameness, and conformation differences are all traits generated by captive breeding but should not be considered complete domestication. The debate is how to differentiate breed from species to categorize small mammals, such as rabbits, ferrets, and many rodents. For the practical purpose of this article, exotic refers to what are often referred to as "nontraditional species"; those patients that are not long-standing within the field of companion veterinary medicine and may include wild or zoologic animals, aquatic species such as fish, relatively common pets such as guinea pigs and parrots, or even domestic animals that have become pets such as chickens, goats, or rabbits. Knowledge of each species' natural histories must guide diagnoses, therapies, husbandry recommendations, socialization techniques, and behavioral management.

Exotic animal medicine and surgery is a rapidly evolving field in veterinary science. Exotic animal medicine and surgery is being regularly taught in veterinary schools and small animal stationary practitioners are seeing exotics at an increased rate.[2,3] Advancements in technology, science, and natural history knowledge have enhanced an understanding of the requirements of these species, allowing earlier diagnoses, interventions, and increasing successful outcomes. Unfortunately, many stationary practicing exotic animal veterinarians practice without the appreciation of ambulatory practice with the insight it can provide. Site-based medicine has great value, as this is where clinical practice can see the answers to questions about the value of natural history. The limitations of this lack of species-specific normal biological understanding may very well lead doctors to treating the symptoms of disease without considering the true etiology.[4]

House calls, farm calls, and site visits to collections have historically provided veterinarians a fundamental understanding of the disease as it relates the husbandry of the group. In bovine, equine, swine, and poultry production medicine, the environment management strategies used through hygiene, sanitation, nutrition, and grouping are central to maximizing production and disease prevention. Exotic ambulatory medicine must have the same principles applied to the species encountered, affecting both individual pets as well as collections. Ambulatory medicine in this article refers to medical care that is provided on a mobile, on-site basis, including consultation, diagnosis, treatment, intervention, and rehabilitation services. Additionally, ambulatory practice includes traveling to the site of the patient or collection to observe them and their dynamic interaction with the environment.

IDENTIFYING THE PROBLEM

The basis of how a captive exotic patient is failing to thrive requires understanding how the animal's captive environment differs from its native environment. Husbandry standards vary, as they are often based on misperceptions of what is an appropriate environment, enclosure, or meal, and can change seasonally based on the given species. Proper assessment of husbandry, whether indoors or outdoors, includes, but is not limited to, the cohabitating species, thermoregulation, humidity, photoregulation, ventilation, microhabitats, toxic plants/insects, nutrition, feed availability, and hygiene/sanitation. Ambulatory practice allows direct observation of diverse animal habitat design giving insight to fundamental health issues.[5–7]

New species are frequently brought to the market as pets.[6] New products, technology, and techniques develop every year. As a result, the practitioner must be responsible for keeping current on the exotic animal marketplace. Personal experience, conversations with colleagues, books, and Internet searches are a few methods of staying current with the market and husbandry. Continuing education is also vital to the process, with the Association of Avian Veterinarians, Association of Exotic Mammal Veterinarians, and Association of Reptilian and Amphibian Veterinarians offering research in medicine, surgery, and exotic animal husbandry.[5,6]

The ability of the exotic animal veterinarian is advanced when understanding of the specific environmental nuance and knowledge gets translated into the reality of replicating functionally important components of the wild habitat.[5,7] The benefits of the lessons learned in ambulatory practice are an integral part of the client education and long-term health of the exotic animal patient. When husbandry needs are met, patients live long enough to need medical interventions that are routinely treated in small animal stationary practice.[7]

Epidemiology is the branch of medicine that deals with the incidence, distribution, possible control of diseases, and other factors relating to health. It is repeated in exotic animal medical literature that disease is largely husbandry/environmentally related. Ambulatory visits are, therefore, the ideal venue for observational interventions for the veterinarian, client education, prevention, and epidemiology (**Fig. 1**).

THE UNION OF FORCES

Good animal health depends on effective communication and teamwork between the veterinarian and the owner/animal steward. Practices can use both ambulatory and stationary services simultaneously, with ambulatory practice providing the best direct observation of the patient's environment. Objective stationary practice knowledge,

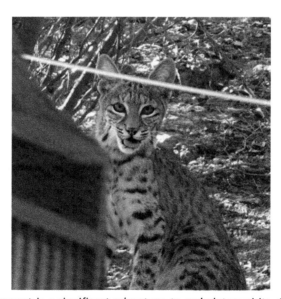

Fig. 1. Risk assessment is a significant advantage to ambulatory visits. Ambulatory visits often give answers to questions that clients do not know to ask. The bobcat in the background was about to attack the African Gray in the cage in the foreground. In addition to predators, other environmental risk factors are either visible or measurable.

unfortunately, is reduced to subjective history gathering about the environment provided. Ambulatory medicine relies on the foundational observation and appropriate environmental interventions to change animal/heard health. In stationary practices, patients commonly arrive without habitat photos or objective environmental data. Stationary practice medicine relies largely on history taking about the basis of the patient's environment from the client's perspective.

Probing questions are necessary for the best possible care. Clients often provide historical information that confirms us of their good intentions but does little to inform/enhance the treatment and well-being of the patient. The standard "What does he/she eat?" question should be replaced with questions of what is offered as well as what is eaten, the portion size, if measured, and how often they are fed. Point in fact is client perception of normal as well as executing captive environments to mirror the function, habitat, and opportunities has to be part of our probing questions. Photos of habitat and food may diminish some of the shortcomings with stationary practice, but rarely do they provide comprehensive environmental understanding.

Holistic health care for the patient is achievable but typically only after reaching veterinary goals and changing client management strategies. Refereed standards of care for most exotic species are not developed or known. Veterinarians should shoulder the responsibility of formulating husbandry plans when species care data are unavailable.

THE DISPARITY OF CARE

Unfortunately, veterinarians are largely more informed about what causes disease as opposed to what promotes health throughout the life of a patient. Clients bring pets/patients into a hospital believing they are providing the best care for their pets. Unlike dog and cat owners, exotic animal owners lack a larger informed community with the same species to compare normal behaviors, diets, habitats, niche, and health. Although the habitat of the (domestic) dog and cat is the shared home of the human, exotic animal habitats in the home can be misperceptions of natural habitat composition in degrees of water, swamp, air, mountains, various forest, desert, and so forth. Exotic animal owners must work harder to comprehend and re-create both habitat and niche of their exotic pet's origin.[4] Clients are often educated through nonprofessionals who simply lack the knowledge of what they don't know. Additionally, veterinary care is usually reactive, as veterinarians are not sought out for preventive medicine or care. A limiting factor in educating clients is getting them to question harmful dogma when they have few questions. Giving framework, perspective, and encouragement to replace dogma when they start to have questions will enhance the life of the patient. The closest to a gold standard for captive habitat and niche are "How does the animal interact and live in the wild?" Most clients have no reasonable "wild context" to understand the disparity in captivity. Exotic animal veterinarians' role is to literally educate the client about the wild animal's evolutionary biology and build the bridge to the captive environment by re-creating its habitat and niche. In summary, if stationary practice is not preceded by ambulatory practice observations/experiences, probing questions of perceived normal habitat, niche, behavior, and husbandry, there are strong limitations on the clinician's ability to assess true health (**Fig. 2**).

Another advantage of ambulatory practice is to help clients understand the disparity between captive/wild behaviors. Psittacines appear to be a group that displays the stress of captivity, as they often display feather destructive behavior despite the client claiming, "The bird has everything it needs." While in captivity, the bird may have food,

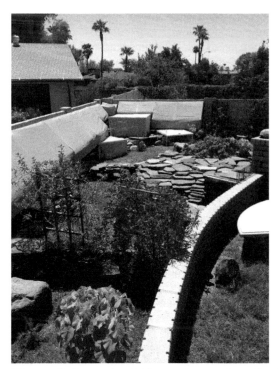

Fig. 2. Shade, humidity, ventilation, and social interactions are but a few benefits of direct visual preventive medicine. The trained veterinarian can help design and alter existing environments through suggestions for best practices for an individual species, such as this desert tortoise habitat. Observing wild tortoise habitats gives key insights to environmental requirements. When combined with available research, appropriate interventions can be advised.

water, shelter, and human attention, it cannot, however, choose its food, activities, flock, to fly, or a mate. It does not have the sovereignty of being wild, social habitat, occupy a given niche, and successfully fill its biological desire to reproduce effectively when kept in the average household. Just as in avian species, although we can treat the symptoms through behavior management, we are not working with the cooperation of evolutionary biology of the patient. Failures to address these needs mute the overall responses to an otherwise scientific approach through functional assessment. Ambulatory practice has the potential to evaluate the environment and work to incorporate changes, social structures, and create behavioral plans.

The following terms must be addressed in an on-site visit to evaluate psychological assessments in exotic animal species:

- *Social parameters* include but are not limited to personality/behavior/sex differences in a single species, behavior changes associated with combinations of species, and niche competition.
- *Social variability* between species is obvious, but interspecies variability is poorly defined and may have individual degrees of expression.
- *Social stressors* both by absence or presence of social enrichment should always be evaluated. If expressed behavior can be quantified, it may be difficult to determine the meaning/value of the expressed behavior and impossible to know

patient thoughts. The ill-defined social parameters create a need to quantify behavior by observable means.

- *Applied behavior analysis* using functional assessment is an effective method to modify and shape behavior. Although this topic is beyond the scope of this article, the author feels that this method has tangible behavior goals and bridges many gaps in literature for individual patients in dynamic situations despite social circumstance. Behavioral recommendations often require multiple visits, client training, client observations, and interventions over days or weeks.

The justification for an ambulatory practice being the initial point of contact for a patient/client is without question truly valuable for their long-term benefit and therefore for the bottom line of either practice type. Exotic animal veterinarians require diverse sets of skills that rival any other profession. Undoubtedly, stationary practices are part of the "union of forces" and play a valuable role in providing quality health care.

ADDING AMBULATORY SERVICES TO A STATIONARY PRACTICE

To be successful with adding an exotic ambulatory practice into an existing exotic stationary practice various processes need to be taken into consideration. As regulations vary based on location, legal consultations to review applicable state law and local regulations are prudent. Population density and client potential are significant factors when assessing the sustainability of an ambulatory exotic practice.

Depending on the vision statements of the fixed practice, the recommendations that follow may vary in applicability. As clients will continue to have access to an existing exotic stationary practice, the ambulatory practice's goal is to fill a need that is not being met. The vision statement, mission statements, and practical implications should be considered, and cooperation, not competition, needs to be the goal of the organization between the practices and will be mutually beneficial. The following list includes items that should be developed according to the specifics of a practice. They are necessary for a well-functioning relationship between an ambulatory and stationary practice. The existing stationary practice can be either a practice that is adding in its own ambulatory services or it may be a practice that is joining forces with a mobile service that had different ownership.

Factors for beginning an ambulatory exotic animal practice:

- Written vision statement: Developed *vision statements* description of why and how a business is to develop and the clarification of the long-term goals. As goals are reached, the vision statement should be modified and therefore should be considered a living document.
- Mission statement: A *mission statement* provides the interim and short-term steps to reaching the vision and can be considered the who and what of a company. The purpose of this document is to define what a company does for its customers, its owner, and its employees.
- Core values: Written *core values* are the belief system of the organization and are used to assess if a company is taking the right path to achieving company goals. These give concise information that builds leadership for the overall team, as well as self-reflection as it considers ethics and purpose. The goal of this document is to give clarity to the owner(s) and tangible expectations to all team members. If joining practices, the owners should agree on vision, mission, and core values the union before the union is considered. In general, the core values should be something unattainable, such as "to practice the highest-quality medicine,"

rather than a measurable target, such as "to get 1000 clients," as these should promote continual advancement.

- Goals: By establishing written *goals* at the onset of the undertaking, the entire team can see how they play a role in the company. As goals are approached, they need to be continually modified, otherwise the purpose will be diminished. Within this, all goals must be realistic and attainable with effort.

AMBULATORY PRACTICE EFFICIENCY

Ambulatory exotic practice associated with a brick-and-mortar practice requires effective staff communication strategies before scheduling visits to be effective and efficient. Appropriate staff training for scheduling appointments will greatly enhance an on-site visit and sets the tone for the delivery of service and client expectations. Administrative staff should assemble previsit client patient data and, ideally, these should be downloadable forms the client will fill out to engage the process of discussion and scheduling. Location of visit/travel time, necessary equipment, and client goals and expectations all need to be clarified. Information provided should include the specie(s) examined, total number of animals needing examinations, habitats encountered, and any other factors that require specific equipment or knowledge. The client needs to be informed that environmental data recorded before the visit should be available and may provide insight. Estimated costs should be clearly communicated before the visit and deposits are recommended to prevent adversarial situations. All of this previsit communication allows for efficient use of in-field veterinary time and enables time to be spent in paid examinations and environmental evaluation.

Vehicle space requirements demand efficiency. Technology greatly decreases space requirements, as portable printers and laptop computers can provide treatment plans, visit summaries, handouts, and records and therefore improve client communication. An organized plan will improve spatial efficiency in that key equipment and supplies can be readily available for the visit, and materials not used will either be in backup locations or not transported.

During the ambulatory visits, the technician takes on a major role for recording information and assembling a written plan as it is verbalized. Physical examinations, photos, and environment suggestions can be recorded in the medical record by the technician. An educational report card summary with common educational topics (stored in a documents file) can be assembled during the visit in a written "report card" as a summary of diagnosis, goals, and treatments.

Improper communications lead to inefficiencies; appropriate communication will help avoid hidden agendas, decrease risk to staff and public, and help establish policies to avoid unnecessary disruptions in animal care. In addition to taking care of a primary concern for the ambulatory visit, the author has been asked to give impromptu classroom lectures, scout meetings, and neighborhood gatherings for unexpected educational "opportunities" during the 45-minute scheduled visit. Although this is great for public relations, it is not fair to regularly scheduled clients. The "wild goose chase on the back 40" is a reality as well. A good policy is that the animals to be examined should be caught and restrained before the visit, and that clients should have it explained to them that increased time on-site for any reason will incur additional fees.

Safety must be a priority and is experience dependent. Dangerous animals require experience and mentoring. Chemical immobilization open to public viewing is not a recommended practice. Specific guidance is recommended before visiting those animals that can bring bodily harm to you, staff, clients, or others who may be around. Escape paths for the animals and people need to be discussed on-site because of the variable environments that will be encountered. Staff should know your limitations and policies for dangerous/venomous animals and zoonotic diseases to effectively communicate policy.

EVALUATING THE CAPTIVE ENVIRONMENT

Ambulatory practitioners should have a basic understanding of each patient's environmental needs and be able to assess the captive environment for functionality. To optimize health, the ambulatory practitioner should consider, develop, educate, and assess the following:

- Husbandry techniques
  - Bedding, cleanliness, heating/cooling devices, appropriate bowls, limbs, perches, hiding structures, microhabitats within habitat
- Products regarding food procurement
  - Hiding food/encouraging foraging behaviors
- Time occupying functional enrichment (environmental or social)
  - Learning and teaching appropriate interactive times with pet/patient
    - Based on both the client's goals and expanding client's current vision
- Functional assessment training
  - Every animal should be mentally challenged
- Space and movement requirement minimums
  - Exercise/activity
  - Thermoregulation
    - Functional access to heat/cooling
- Photoregulation
  - Functional access to light and UV (distance, hides)
  - Appropriate photoperiod
- Ventilation
  - Environment should have active air movement
- Humidity
  - Must be properly humidified and balanced with appropriate ventilation.

PRACTICAL ADVICE FOR THE AMBULATORY SERVICE

- Merge with an existing practice or rent part of a stationary facility for procedures that will enhance the success of the patient.
  - Find a colleague(s) you can partner with while you grow.
    - Requirements for surgical site
    - Hospitalization requirements
    - Radiology services
  - Define the agreement with the colleague in writing.
    - All clients' dogs and cats can be referred to the colleague?
    - All exotic clients will be referred to ambulatory?
      - As the brick-and-mortar practice, a DVM who works for you must agree to a mutually beneficial, enforceable, noncompete clause.
- When starting an exotics ambulatory, start small and grow. Pay the bills and needed salary and expand as it is practical.
  - May need to "moonlight" or work relief initially to provide sufficient income.
  - Do not overspend on equipment initially.

- ○ Space is a premium in an ambulatory service. Add equipment if practical to carry when likely to be financially successful.
- Knowledge is the most valuable asset for patient care.
  - ○ Environmental disease prevention requires species-specific knowledge (habitat and patient) and practical husbandry abilities to be manipulated consistent with patient natural history.
  - ○ Specific behavior knowledge and the ability to create positive changes, appropriate interventions, and displacement are important.
- Ambulatory practices give as much insight about the animal steward (owner/caretaker) as the animal and the environments. Compassion for financial limitations may unconsciously influence the quality of medicine being offered.
  - ○ Hygiene and sanitation are not optional practices.
  - ○ Best veterinary medicine is our obligation for the patient.
- Ambulatory client relationships foster deep personal relationships and loyalty through connections built at visits.
- During the house call, be aware of potential adverse events.
  - ○ Avoid disaster by inquiring about patient escape or interfering people/dog/cats, as well as open doors, ceiling fans, and other hazards that patients may encounter.
  - ○ Consider capture myopathy and habitat hygiene.
  - ○ The plan, order of operations, and appropriate hygiene all demonstrate good medicine and provide an example for the owner.
- Be mindful of being a fomite for disease. Handwashing and appropriate clean equipment, and personal protective equipment (gowns, foot covers, mask, gloves, and face shields) should be used.
- It is not worthwhile to attempt to capture injured wildlife that cannot be contained or fenced before arrival. Leave that for the professionals.
- The best interest of the patient should be the primary interest.
  - ○ Is ambulatory or stationary practice care best?
  - ○ Which would be the least traumatic with the best benefit?
- When in doubt, refer to vision and mission. Decisions should be made the reflect vision and mission statements and align with your core values.

THE PRACTITIONER WHO WILL LEAD THE SERVICE

- Should be relationship oriented without compromising patient advocacy
- Must be a critical thinker and problem solver
- Research before and after visit to resolve best solution
- Must be pragmatic in the field
- Must be prepared for trial and error

GROWTH INTO A STATIONARY PRACTICE

Veterinarians who decide to start their own practice often test the viability of exotic animal medicine for the advantages of a low start-up cost and flexibility. The long-term goals may include opening up a stationary practice as finances permit. "Growth pains" are a given and are particularly difficult when trying to provide the patient/client the benefits of both practice types as a solo practitioner.

The advantages of an exotic ambulatory practice are notable. Low overhead cost as a start-up is a large initial advantage. It is more affordable and convenient for larger collections of animals in which heard health is most crucial. The focus of achieving health to the individual and/or group is the goal of both ambulatory and stationary practice. The method used to achieve the focus health is direct observation/routine medicine as opposed to history taking through veterinary questioning to owners who may not be aware of what valid concerns may be.

At the same time, there are advantages of a stationary exotic practice when it relates to readily available diagnostic modalities, controlled surgical environments, emergency services, and specialized hospitalization. The offices can be structured to educate owners with literature, videos, and computers. Additionally, more clients can be seen in a shorter period of time.

When a practice merges with or adds a "brick-and-mortar" to the ambulatory service and is large enough to support additional practitioners, effective written medical record communication and client-provided habitat photos become vital for the understanding of those practitioners. Visual quantifiable and visual intuitive information (nonquantifiable) inform decisions made regarding "environmental disease" in the ambulatory practice that are difficult to convey in office settings. It is a best practice to have clients bring in photographs when ambulatory calls are not possible to assess the habitat at least in a visual sense. Photos should be labeled with habitat orientation with outdoor environments so seasonal extremes can be meliorated.

Defining the scope of what can and should be done in both practice types is species-specific and creates a lot of questions from front office staff. Hiring staff who can solve problems, not staff who just know the rules, is imperative to a well-functioning business. Office staff should take a lead role at discussing the benefits of an ambulatory visit at the same time as to consider financial concerns from the owner. Although training is helpful, many variables create further staff/client questions.

The inevitable outcome of good management of a mobile practice is that patient retention is longer, which is good for the clients, patients, and profitability. The reality for a well-managed ambulatory practice is that it is difficult over time to keep up with ambulatory practices because of patient volume and demand. It is at that point worth reviewing goals and reassessing vision. If hiring another veterinarian is financially viable and aligns with the mission statement, it should be done. Although transitioning and mentoring can have difficulties, it is also rewarding and legacy-minded. When starting the stationary practice, the ambulatory practice should be maintained to provide income and allows the associate to develop necessary skills and insight for disease at the level of environment disease. Discontinuing an ambulatory practice will result in client loss for those who require the service due to patient size or herd/flock size, or who have disabilities that preclude driving.

The well-managed ambulatory practice builds a foundation of medical expertise that gives the stationary practitioner insight through diverse experiences.

- Expertise is developed in the ability to make necessary manipulations in the local climate to meet the biological needs of the patients.
- Expertise is developed in comprehending various social interactions and adaptive behaviors in artificial environments.
- Expertise is developed through diverse collections and diverse environments.
- Expertise develops because diagnosis exists without the dependence of incomplete client perceptions of health.
- Expertise develops because hygiene and sanitation practices are observable.

SUMMARY

Incorporating ambulatory medicine into a brick-and-mortar practice is perhaps the most valuable component to expansion of the field by insight to creating health in addition to treating preventable husbandry-related disease. Each practice type done individually is incomplete and has complementary advantages and disadvantages. Together they lend valuable insights to cause effective treatment. Ambulatory services can provide major advantages when patient size and number; behavior-related problems; nutrition; and herd, flock, or group medical management need to be addressed. Environmental assessments (design, flow, best practices, hygiene, sanitation, disinfection, thermoregulation, photo regulation, predator avoidance, environmental disturbances, toxic plants, and humidity) are also better assessed by direct visualization afforded by ambulatory care. As nontraditional medicine is one of the most rapidly developing fields of veterinary care, it is critical to provide the best possible assessments so that we do not lose perspective of the purpose. Environment-related disease assessments in a stationary practice are largely dependent on the subjective, overlooked, and underappreciated historical details given by the animal's stewards.

The goal of growing into a stationary practice can be a worthwhile direction. In addition, maintaining an ambulatory practice as a part of the stationary practice adds tools and insight that cannot be readily duplicated by other methodology. When addressing a pathologic condition, simply treating the disease is less effective than preventing it, facilitated through the direct observational advantage of an ambulatory practice.

Ambulatory practice is personally engaging, requires critical thinking, and fosters incredible loyalty. Merging mobile and stationary practice with the insight advantage is a good compromise and allows for the best possible medicine to be practiced. The union of forces necessary for exotic animal medicine is both ambulatory and stationary practice, as it benefits the most patients in this developing field. Because it combines the knowledge of the patient in its environment with appropriate medical diagnostics to achieve the medical understanding, we are able to accomplish a level of holistic care unlike any other time is history.

The best interest of the patient is the only interest to be considered, and in order that the sick may have the benefit of advancing knowledge, union of forces is necessary.

—*William J. Mayo, MD, 1910.*

REFERENCES

1. Available at: http://www.dictionary.com/browse/domestic-animal.
2. Available at: https://www.veterinarianedu.org/exotic-animal-vet/.
3. Pollock CG. Survey on avian medical education in US veterinary colleges (2002–2004). J Avian Med Surg 2004;18:183–8.
4. Doneley Robert JT. Ten things I wish I'd learned at university. Vet Clin North Am Exot Anim Pract 2005;8(3):393–404.
5. Bradley Bays T. Equipping the reptile practice. Vet Clin North Am Exot Anim Pract 2005;8(3):437–61.
6. Mayer J, Martin J. Barriers to exotic animal medicine. Vet Clin North Am Exot Anim Pract 2005;8(3):487–96.
7. Driggers T. The mobile exotic pet practice. Vet Clin North Am Exot Anim Pract 2005;8(3):463–8.

Ambulatory Exotic Animal Medicine Legal Issues

Adolf K. Maas III, DVM, CertAqVet, DABVP (Reptile and Amphibian Medicine and Surgery)[a,b,*]

KEYWORDS

- Liability • Exotic animals • Legal issues • Law • Off-label • Accreditation • Risk
- Jurisdiction

KEY POINTS

- Ambulatory exotic animal practice shares many of the legal concerns as stationary practices, but also has unique issues that need to be addressed.
- Ambulatory practitioners must be familiar with federal and local codes and regulations, and must recognize that regulations may vary in different areas of their practice range.
- Unique liability issues are presented with ambulatory nontraditional species practice but are mitigated with good planning.
- It is the responsibility of the practitioner to research, learn, and understand the laws, codes, and regulations that may affect them: "Ignorance of the law is no excuse."

INTRODUCTION

Ambulatory veterinary practice is similar to stationary veterinary practice in that it deals with the diagnosis, prevention, and treatment of animal diseases. The primary difference is that rather than having the patient come to the practitioner, the practitioner comes to the patient. When addressing nontraditional animal species, there are many similarities to companion animal medicine; however the techniques and diagnoses can change dramatically.

Legal issues in ambulatory medicine of exotic animal species bring additional regulations ranging from pharmaceutical and animal transport to legalities and regulations of possessing or treating particular species, and even to the therapeutic options available. Many of these concerns are extensions of those designed for domestic animals with additional legal implications and ethical responsibilities of the practitioner.

The implications and responsibilities fit into three primary sections: (1) regulations concerning exotic animal possession and treatment originating from jurisdictional laws, (2) legal issues concerning the exotic animal practitioner originating from a medical perspective, and (3) legal matters that relate to liability and injury. Whereas many

Disclosure: The author has nothing to disclose.
[a] Toledo Zoo, 2 Hippo Drive, Toledo, Ohio 43614, USA; [b] ZooVet Consulting, PLLC, PO Box 1007, Bothell, WA 98041, USA
* ZooVet Consulting, PLLC, PO Box 1007, Bothell, WA 98041.
E-mail address: DrMaas@zoovet.us

vetexotic.theclinics.com

of these limitations and issues have counterparts in domestic stationary and ambulatory animal practice, there are additional factors that must be considered.

This article provides an overview of available legislation that is pertinent to the ambulatory exotic animal practice and a summary of currently accepted guidelines for which there is often no official statute. It is not to be construed as an all-inclusive summary of exotic animal laws and legislation. Neither is it to be deemed legal advice or replacement for legal counsel.

REGULATIONS

In every part of the United States, there are legal regulations that apply to animal possession and veterinary medicine. These laws are divided into federal and local jurisdictional regulations. It is important to understand that although these may not always be in agreement with each other, there is a hierarchy as to their regulation.

Although federal laws must be obeyed, at a minimum each progressively smaller municipality has the authority to enact/adopt more stringent laws or regulations, but cannot make regulations that are less stringent than the next larger district. This is analogous to taxation: the federal government has established and maintains a federal tax statute that determines that amount of tax every person and entity must pay each year. Each state subsequently establishes the tax level that they choose to assess the resident population and businesses. From there, counties, cities, townships, and districts each assess their own taxes. At the same time, no state or municipality can eliminate federal taxation in favor of its own rules and regulations, just as a county cannot eliminate a state's taxation, and so on. Whereas, say a county, has the option to assess no taxation, it also does not have the authority to eliminate the requirement of a person to pay state or federal taxes. In short, any municipality included within the larger political jurisdiction has the authority to place further burdens (increase regulation) but not the authority to reduce the limitations placed by the larger entity. Such are the laws concerning exotic animals.

It is critical for an ambulatory exotic animal clinician to be familiar with the regulations of all the areas that they service, including the states and counties that they operate within and any cities/town and districts they provide service to. "*Ignorantia juris non excusat*," or "Ignorance of the law excuses not," is an almost universal theme in modern Western law, well represented in case law for more than 200 years. Although there are exceptions to this rule, the courts generally do not accept ignorance of the law as a viable excuse for breaching these hard-to-locate regulations, particularly in veterinary medicine where each state clearly specifies that each practitioner is responsible for following the practice code and regulations as a preclude to licensure. Therefore, it is the veterinarian's responsibility to know whether or not they can legally treat a given animal and to advise a client on how to proceed. It is emphatically recommended that the person claiming responsibility for an animal contact the appropriate authorities for specific information regarding the particular species if there is any ambiguity or question of legality. It should also be noted that substantially all municipal employees are not authorized to give legal advice. Any advice by them on which one may rely should be obtained from them on official stationery in writing or personally verified before acting in reliance thereon and potentially subjecting the clinician to consequences.

Regrettably, there is no single resource listing either all of the state's laws/regulations or even all of the controlling statutes within a given state. However, most states and municipalities provide access to their codes via the Internet. The problem is that the codes are often difficult to locate, particularly for the less populous or smaller municipalities.

REGULATIONS CONCERNING THE PRACTICE OF EXOTIC ANIMAL MEDICINE
Federal Legal Issues

The federal government provides the basis of many of the laws that are encountered, but these laws are now only a subset of the regulations that may be faced. These regulations, as previously discussed, are universal and violation of these can cause significant impositions on the practitioner. The primary areas of federal regulation that affect an ambulatory exotic animal practitioner are divided into regulations regarding the transport and care of animals, the administration of pharmacotherapeutics and biologics in animals, and the storage and transport of controlled substances.

Convention on the International Trade of Endangered Species, the Lacey Act, and the Marine Mammal Protection Act

The federal government regulates transport of conserved, threatened, and endangered species of animals across international and interstate borders. Although ambulatory practitioners only uncommonly encounter situations where these apply, it is important to understand the implications of these regulations.

The Convention on the International Trade of Endangered Species (CITES) was designed to control and regulate the movement of animal species at risk of damage in their indigenous territory. In addition to the prevention of extirpation of these animals by capture and sale into the private sector, it is also designed to hamper/halt the trade of body parts or materials obtained through poaching or other illegal methods. This can affect the exotic animal practitioner in three more common aspects, discussed next.

International health certificates for the relocation of pets or zoologic species It is not uncommon in today's world for people to relocate internationally, even if only from the United States to Canada or Mexico. Because they likely relocate with their pets, animals that are legally obtained in the United States require CITES permits to be transported.[1] This is especially common with pet bird species that are often recognized as threatened or endangered in the wild. Zoologic species in collections almost always require a CITES permit, and whereas American Zoological Association-accredited facilities have programs in place to facilitate moves of animals into or from the collection, many small private zoos and facilities do not and rely on their veterinarian to assemble the paperwork.

When tasked with providing permits to transport any exotic species out of the United States, it is absolutely critical that the owner first be advised of the time frame that may be necessary to obtain the required permits. Additionally, the country of importation needs to be directly contacted to acquire the specific current requirements of the species being transported, including documentation of the individual, required vaccinations and pathologic testing, and to be certain of the time frame during which all of this needs to be performed. Based on personal experience, the author strongly recommends that the practitioner advise the client to retain the services of a professional international animal transport service.

CITES also affects exotic animal practitioners in that it limits the transport of tissue, fluids, or cutaneous samples across international borders. Again, affecting a clinician little, a CITES permit is required to ship blood, tissue, feathers, or similar samples from registered species into or out of the United States. If a clinician needs to ship samples for research, diagnosis, or other purposes across national borders, inquiries as to CITES status and availability of permits are necessary.

Interstate transport of US native species The Lacey Act, as it relates to practitioners, regulates the transport of native endangered species across state lines and prevents the introduction of deleterious species into new territories. The best-known example of deleterious species is the Brown Tree snake (*Boiga irregularis*), which is native to Southeast Asia. This snake has been the cause of the extinction of several species of birds in Guam and surrounding islands, and has brought many other species of birds and bats to endangerment where the snake has been introduced outside of its native range. Because this species is remarkably (and initially unexpected) adaptable to a wide range of environments, there is real concern that if introduced to the US mainland, it would have a drastic deleterious effect on much of the western hemisphere. Thus, this species is strictly forbidden on US territories.

Whereas few other species have the limitations of Brown Tree snakes, the transport of many species across state lines require permits or are prohibited all together. Although there are regulations regarding the transport of species not on protection lists, any native species that is deemed endangered within the United States borders requires permits to transport across state lines. The Indigo snake (*Drymarchon couperi*) is one such example, because it is native to the Southeastern United States and has protective status. Although it is captive bred and privately possessed in almost all states, transport of these animals from one state to another requires a permit under the Lacey Act. Many other species of animals also require these permits.

Wildlife interactions Exotic animal practitioners commonly perform treatment on wildlife species; ambulatory practitioners regularly encounter injured or ill animals and are asked to provide (at least emergency) treatment. In addition to state laws, there are federal regulations that can affect the mobile veterinarian. The Migratory Bird Act requires that all persons involved in the care or rehabilitation of wildlife must possess a valid migratory bird permit or be an approved subpermittee of a permit holder. A subset of the Migratory Bird Act also regulates the possession, ownership, and care of birds of prey used in falconry. The Migratory Bird Act and the Lacey Act and the Animal Welfare Act regulate transportation of falconry birds across state boundaries. Violation of any or all of these can result in jail time and severe penalties.

The Marine Mammal Protection Act applies to all species of mammals that live in marine environments. Although there are many other regulations within this act, it is critical for all exotic animal veterinarians to remember that it is strictly prohibited to "to hunt, harass, capture, or kill any marine mammal or attempt to do so"[2] and strictly prohibits coming within 100 yards (or more, depending on species) of any whale or 50 yards of any seal, sea lion, or porpoise or dolphin (more in some locations).[3] Any animal found that seems to need medical attention must be reported to the US Fish and Wildlife Service before it is approached, handled, or treated, and in most cases, the US Fish and Wildlife Service dispatches agents to attend to the needs of these animals rather than have private practitioners attempt to do so.

US Department of Agriculture/Food and Drug Administration
The United States Department of Agriculture (USDA) and the Food and Drug Administration have three primary areas of regulation that affect the ambulatory nontraditional animal practitioner. The first of these involves pharmaceutical use and drug residues in the animals administered. Although they may be considered pets and never enter into the food chain, nontraditional species, such as rabbits, chickens, ducks, goats, zebu, and dwarf cattle, plus any wildlife species, must never receive any banned pharmacology agents, such as aminoglycosides and fluoroquinolones. Any drugs that are not banned but are not specifically approved by the USDA must

have withdrawal times established and presented to the owner as part of the treatment plan. Any drug that does not have a formal withdrawal time needs to be assessed by the Food Animal Residue Avoidance and Databank and, based on the drug, dose, species, and size of the animal a recommended withdrawal time is recommended. This step is critical not only to prevent legal liability on the practitioner but also to avert serious violations the USDA regulations.

The second area of USDA/Food and Drug Administration regulation that the exotic animal practitioner is affected by involves off-label administration of therapeutics to the species seen. In most cases there are no approved pharmaceuticals for the animal being treated, thus other standards have been accepted within the exotic veterinary community. Where a clinician is to treat an animal with a drug that they have not commonly used in that species, the practitioner must rely on the three basic rules of zoologic clinical pharmacology[4] and common sense:

1. The doctor should make reasonable investigation to determine what she or he can about the function, adverse reactions, risks, pharmacokinetics, and disposition of that drug as known in other species.
2. Contact should be made with individuals known to or reasonably believed to have experience with that particular drug in the species intended, or at least in a closely related species.
3. If no record has been found of use of that drug in the species to be treated, use with extreme caution. Never use the drug in cases where an animal cannot be lost as a result of adverse effects or reactions.

It is only prudent to add this fourth rule to the repertoire:

4. Before proceeding with the administration of the any extralabel drug, the veterinarian must explain the risks and the potential benefits of the particular medication to the owner. After the pros and cons have been thoroughly explained, it is necessary for the veterinarian to prepare a written release that acknowledges that the drugs/therapies being administered are "off-label." The client must sign it, acknowledging the risks and authorizing the veterinarian to proceed with the proposed treatment. It is the sole responsibility of the veterinarian to present all adverse reactions of the therapy being administered. Anything less is inviting a lawsuit for damages or unprofessional conduct because of lack of full disclosure. Federal law requires veterinarians to maintain a record of all extralabel drug use, including justification for its application, for a minimum of 2 years. These records and the signed release may be maintained in the regular medical record, but the practitioner is responsible for knowing the retention regulations of the states in which they practice. A sample form is demonstrated in **Fig. 1**.

When it comes to the treatment of amphibians and fish, there is a potential that many of the drugs commonly used are excreted in a functional form into the environment in which they live. This can have significant effects on their health and the health of tank mates and beneficial microbes. This aspect must be seriously considered before administration.

The Minor Use in Minor Species Animal Health Act, having been passed in 2004, makes the use of pharmaceuticals in the practice of exotic animal medicine much less uncertain. This act allows conditional approval for drugs to be used in less well-studied species (ie, wildlife, exotics) when there has been demonstrated a reasonable level of safety and efficacy. Additionally, for species where it is not economically feasible to conduct even conditional approval studies, there is a list of

All prescription drugs (pharmaceuticals, or "legend drugs") are regulated by the FDA, and to be released for sale and use, must be approved for specific use in designated species and for particular treatment and protocols. To be approved, every drug must go through a series of testing and analysis to understand not only the benefits and effects, but also the side-effects and risks of its use. This must be repeated extensively in each species for which the medication's use is to be approved in.

This process for FDA approval is very expensive and the manufacturers traditionally pursue approval for species in which they expect to have sufficient sales to be able to recoup their expenses. These typically include dogs and cats, and, in some medications, horses, cows, pigs and occasionally a few other domesticated species. At this time, very few pharmaceuticals are approved in fish, rats and rabbits, while no drug or medication is approved for use in any pet bird, reptile, or most small exotic mammals.

Use of pharmaceuticals in species for which they are not approved is allowed, however, and is termed "Extra-Label Use". This does not mean that the use is experimental, and in many cases years of clinical use and research has found a well-documented, reasonably safe protocol for the use of these medications in species for which no other medical option is available. However, "Extra-Label Use" does mean that the full effect and side effects of the drug have not been documented and there may be unknown risks involved with the use of the medication in intested species.

ZooVet Consulting, PLLC prides itself in striving to provide the highest level of medicine available to your bird, reptile, small mammal, fish or other exotic pet. Virtually all of the medications administered by ZooVet Consulting, PLLC fall under the "extra-label use" category and the protocols prescribed have basis in either clinical experience or published reports. If you have any questions regarding any medication or therapy recommended by Dr. Maas, please feel comfortable to discuss these at any time.

The undersigned acknowledges that Extra-Label Use of pharmaceuticals is acceptable therapy to be used in their pet or animal, as deemed necessary by the attending veterinarian and that they approve prescriptions to be made and filled. The owner understands that although all reasonable precautions will be taken to minimize or mitigate adverse effects, there are risks inherent to any pharmaceutical use in exotic and non-traditional medicine.

_____   _____

Owner's Signature   Date

_____

Printed Name

Fig. 1. Exotic animal pharmaceuticals. (*Courtesy of* ZooVet Consulting, PLLC, Bothell, WA; with permission.)

"index drugs" that are legal for conditional approval and use. In short, the Minor Use in Minor Species Animal Health Act provides a legal basis for the use of drugs within the exotic pet practice, and removes at least some of the concerns with extralabel drug use.[5]

The last area of interaction between the USDA and the ambulatory exotic animal practitioner involves accreditation of the practitioner. It is important to remember that USDA accreditation is awarded on a state-by-state basis and that there is no reciprocity or "carryover" from one state to another, no matter which states the practitioner holds a license to practice veterinary medicine. With type 1 accreditation being specific only for doctors practicing medicine limited to dogs and cats, the nontraditional species practitioner must have type 2 accreditation to provide health certificates or inspections to facilities requiring USDA certificates. The reader is recommended to refer to the Susan Horton's article, "USDA Facility Inspection for Exotic Veterinarians," in this issue. If the veterinarian travels over state lines as part of their range, it is necessary for them to obtain accreditation in each state in which they practice. Further information is obtained at https://www.usda.gov.

Drug Enforcement Agency

The Drug Enforcement Agency regulates the distribution/diversion and transport of controlled drugs within the United States. Any ambulatory practitioner purchasing, using, administering, or carrying scheduled therapeutics is required to obtain and carry a Controlled Substance Registration Certificate at all times. Recent regulations have changed the rules concerning the carrying and transport of scheduled drugs,[6] and the specifics of amounts of each type of drug that is allowed to be transported, so although it is legal for ambulatory veterinarians to retain these compounds with them in their practice, it is strongly advised that each doctor review current regulations annually to be certain to be within approved laws. Although there is a well-established Web site (https://www.deadiversion.usdoj.gov/) it is often necessary to inquire with an agent to get the necessary information.

Jurisdictional Legal Issues

Although the federal regulations are uniform, there are few federal laws concerning the practice of veterinary medicine. Each state (with instances of county, municipality, and city regulations) has enacted codes that define the responsibilities and duties of veterinarians, laws concerning possession and ownership, and treatment of animals. Some states are even instituting laws that define the rights of animals. The following are some of the more commonly encountered regulations that need to be addressed as an ambulatory exotic animal practitioner, but it is advised that every veterinarian review the specifics of their practicing range.

Veterinary Practice Act

The Veterinary Practice Act (VPA) is an organized collection of rules, unique to each state, that provides the codes and regulations that every clinician is required to have full knowledge of and understand to practice within that state. Each state's VPA specifies the minimum standards of veterinary medicine to be practiced within that state, often with definitions specifying differences between "large animal" and "small animal" medicine, and most states now define the minimum provisions for stationary and ambulatory practices. All of these apply to the mobile exotic animal practitioner, plus many states now require registry for mobile practices just as for stationary practices. This means that in addition to defined standards, rules, and regulations, mobile practices are reviewed and inspected regularly, and may have additional fees and taxes imposed, depending on jurisdiction. Most states no longer require a clinical competency examination to gain licensure, whereas almost all states require a Juris Prudence examination testing every incoming clinician on their familiarity with the rules and regulations of that territory.

Because most states require that mobile practices have availability of radiology services, this can require that either a mobile radiology unit and ancillary equipment be carried or that the practitioner have an arrangement with a stationary practice for at least the purpose of taking radiographs at their facility. Additionally, some states require that formal agreements be made for purposes of hospitalization and/or emergency services. It is advised that the ambulatory exotics practitioner assemble written agreements with "brick and mortar" practices for the services required in their states, keeping in mind that several arrangements may be necessary to provide appropriate services in their travel area. Copies of these written agreements should be retained within the practice vehicle so that they can be presented on demand as needed.

Veterinary-client-patient relationship

All states require the formation of a valid veterinary-client-patient relationship (VCPR) to be able to provide therapy to a patient, and the VCPR is no less important because it may not be a dog or cat. Although the requirements of a valid VCPR vary from state to state, there are six principles established by the American Veterinary Medical Association (AVMA) that are uniform in all definitions:

- Maintain written agreements for working relationships
- Have a veterinarian of record
- Clarify any and all relationships with consultants and other veterinarians
- Provide written protocols
- Ensure written or electronic treatment records are maintained
- Provide drugs or prescriptions for specific time frames and for specific protocols

If these principles are met, the practitioner will meet all or nearly all requirements in every state, although each state may define these principles differently. For example, the State of Washington requires that all prescription labels be typed for clarity, whereas Montana allows prescription labels to be hand written. Thus, it is entirely up to the clinician to research and follow the regulations appropriate for the region that they are practicing in and to follow the standards established in each jurisdiction.

Record keeping

Proper record keeping is a significant part of meeting the VCPR guidelines and critical for practicing good medicine. As an ambulatory practitioner, this means that all records must be accessible at each site visited. Again, each state's requirements for typed versus hand-written records are different and are rapidly changing, so it is important to check with the regulations in each jurisdiction. One advantage is that veterinarians are not required (at this time) to follow HIPAA-level security so that with the combination of laptop computers, portable "hot-spots," and on-line records storage ("cloud" computing) the burden of proper record keeping is easily met with current technology.

Permitted species

Just as each state has their own regulations concerning the VCPR and record keeping, each state has set specific laws and regulations concerning what species are allowed within their borders. The federal regulations (mostly within the CITES regulations and the acts described previously) are in effect in all states and territories, whereas the smaller jurisdictions each have the right to enforce additional restrictions, as the constituents deem appropriate.

As a result, one of the most common issues faced by exotic animal practitioners is addressing possession of prohibited nontraditional species, including wildlife. It is not uncommon for a client to present an injured or ill wild animal species for treatment and not have the legal right to possess it. This animal may or may not be designated as a pet and may or may not have been obtained legally. The following questions should arise in each of these situations:

- What should be done if the client requests that the animal be returned after consultation?
- Should the animal be refused treatment, even if such refusal would most likely result in that animal's suffering or death?
- Should the animal be returned to the client if the client has agreed to pay for the treatment if and only if the animal is returned to them following treatment?
- Is the veterinarian required to treat and then transfer an injured animal along to a wildlife rehabilitator, risking alienation of the client?

These are questions that are as much ethical as legal, and must be determined by the clinician based on factors they deem relevant and applicable to the laws of their jurisdiction.

If the decision is for the animal to be treated and returned, the clients should be notified that the veterinarian may be obligated to contact appropriate authorities to advise them of the possessors' infraction and situation, which may relieve the clinician of some liability. States have varying guidelines and codes concerning possession of native species. If there is any uncertainty regarding the guidelines and statutes for a practitioner's jurisdiction, the local and state governing agencies should be contacted. There is no federal regulation that a veterinarian must treat all cases presented to them (even if the doctor also holds appropriate wildlife rehabilitation permits) any more than a traditional pet practice is required to accept all pets that enter their facility as patients.

To consider an alternative, assume that instead of a wildlife species, the animal in question is a ferret, residing in a "ferret-free zone." In some states, the law implies that veterinarians treating illegally possessed animals may be deemed to be "aiding and abetting a known criminal." By violating this law, veterinarians may be subjecting themselves to sanctions up to and including the possible loss of their license to practice. Other jurisdictions permit veterinarians to treat the animal, putting the welfare of the animal first and considering the owner's infraction a separate issue. This situation further illustrates the need to review the local jurisdictional guidelines.

Liability Legal Issues

In addition to federal, state, and local regulations, there are state and municipality codes that assess the practice of veterinary medicine. These are likely the legal issues that the ambulatory practitioner will encounter regularly and should be aware of at all times, in every case. Malpractice and liability insurance should be carried by each practice and practitioner for these reasons, but insurance should never be a justification for neglect.

Off-label issues

There are federal regulations concerning off-label administration of therapeutics, but there are also liabilities to the practitioner for prescribing. Because most of the risks involve level of communication, the simplest way to avoid liability is to provide as complete of disclosure as possible. It is important to have all clients agree to and sign acknowledgments of off-label pharmaceutical administration, but even more so to inform the client of basic risks with each therapeutic. Advising them that if they would like more detailed information and discussions they are available at any point in the treatment plan also mitigates the liability to the practitioner.

Standards of care

Even though there are few approved drugs and even fewer established therapies, there is still a standard of care that is expected from every veterinarian, in every case, and in every species. In most states, the jurisdictional VPA defines at least part of this, but the state's veterinary practice board defines the actual standards.[7] It is important to remember that in no case does the value of an animal or the owner's ability/willingness to pay for services establish the standard of care, but rather what is considered to be an appropriate level based on current published standards.

To prevent legal liability for not providing the standard of care the doctor must assess their levels of skills and knowledge, because all states are clear that when a clinician exceeds their training and abilities, they are wholly liable for any complications and problems. At the same time, if the clinician selects a treatment plan that is less than then standard of care to, say, accommodate the wishes of the owner's budget, the clinician is also liable for failure of success, complications, or other problem. To reduce or relieve the veterinarian of risk of malpractice, it is strongly recommended that the clinician clearly explain the differences in therapy between the standard of care and the therapy chosen by the client, the risk of complications and failure, and to have the owner sign and date a form informing the client that they, rather than the doctor, are choosing the treatment. These are often referred to as "against doctor's recommendations" forms and should be written specifically to address the VPA of that state, and then incorporated into the permanent medical record of that patient. To help resolve these issues, some states have passed regulations; Wisconsin, for example, has a code within their VPA that requires clinicians present all known treatment options to every patient in every case, including the options of referral and euthanasia.

In recognizing one's limitations (whether it be of a species, disease, treatment plan, or those imposed by being an ambulatory practitioner), it is critical that every mobile nontraditional species veterinarian establish a resource base for which to send patients on referral.[8] Not only does this reduce the risk of liability by transferring cases that one is not skilled in treating, it provides a venue to reduce liability when the owners choose not to pursue referral services. Again, documentation is critical in these situations and at a minimum notes should be included in the patient's permanent record.

Anesthesia/surgical risks

Although there are always risks associated with anesthesia, working on nontraditional species adds another level of concern and liability. Other than for fish, there are no approved anesthetic agents or protocols for any of these species, in addition to concerns about drug residue and poorly understood physiology of anesthesia in most species. To mitigate the liability faced by a veterinarian in these patients, off-label, USDA/Food Animal Residue Avoidance and Databank, and standard of care issues must all be addressed in advance with the client and documentation of all approvals and discussions kept within the patient's permanent chart as required by the state's VPA.

To further compound matters, anesthesia and surgery have additional risks when performed on a mobile basis. The risk of contamination, poor lighting, inadequate materials, equipment, and environment for recovery are some of the concerns, with more added based on the exact situation, condition, and patient being dealt with. The easiest way to reduce liability involves two aspects. First, provide the same level of anesthesia and surgery as would be performed in a stationary practice, except at the site if necessary. Mobile anesthetic units are now commonly available, as are surgical ventilators. Any equipment that is routinely used in a stationary practice is available as a portable, battery powered unit, including fluid pumps, electrocardiograms, blood pressure monitors, pulse oximetry units, ultrasound units, and endoscopy setups. Just as one would invest and use these in a stationary practice, all of these should be used the same in an ambulatory practice.

Most, if not all, VPAs require the use of heat- or gas-sterilized instrumentation, and providing clean fields and drapes. The simple addition of LED head lamps and loupes improves lighting in any situation, and for all but perhaps the most invasive of orthopedic procedures, the standard of care can be met in the confines of a fully mobile practice.

Second, communicate clearly with the client to establish reasonable limitations, expectations, and risk factors. Not only does complete communication and documentation dramatically reduce liability, but it allows the practitioner a good understanding of what the owner's expectations are and permits an assessment for whether or not the clinician can meet these expectations. Well-written anesthesia and surgical permission forms specific to exotic animal ambulatory medicine assist with the communication and spell out standard risk factors for the client. According to the American Veterinary Medical Association - Professional Liability Insurance Trust (AVMA-PLIT) (John Schedler, AVMA PLIT attorney, personal communication, 2015), most surgical/anesthesia malpractice claims could have been prevented or dismissed if the attending veterinarian had provided clear communication and documented it within the patient record.

Bailment

Bailment in veterinary medicine is defined is the act of transporting animals to or from a setting, usually to a veterinary clinic or to an owner's house. When vehicular accidents occur or trauma or death happen while an animal is being transported, the veterinarian/veterinary practice is legally liable.[9] It is important to know that neither automobile liability insurance nor malpractice insurance provide coverage for these events, and most business insurance specifically excludes bailment coverage. Because bailment insurance is inexpensive through most personal liability insurance providers (ie, AVMA PLIT) it is advised that every ambulatory practitioner add this to their coverage. Although umbrella liability policies also do not typically cover bailment, if a practitioner has already added bailment insurance to their policy, most umbrella policies then cover liabilities beyond the limits of the bailment policy. Conversations with licensed insurance representatives should be able to provide the information necessary to make appropriate decisions.

"Good Samaritan" laws

One additional reference to the treatment of wildlife and prohibited/permitted species is each jurisdiction's laws concerning immediate, necessary treatment of injured and sick animals. Many VPAs have provisions for veterinarians to provide emergency care and stabilization of animals that they otherwise may not be authorized, qualified, or licensed to treat. More specifically, these codes provide legal protection to the attending doctor for liability that they may incur by providing assistance, even if the animal is not legal in that jurisdiction or if the veterinarian does not have proper licensure to work on that animal, so long as there is not remuneration for the services provided. The primary exception to these laws involves marine mammals, because the federal law takes precedence and is the most stringent, prohibiting anyone without specific federal permission to contact a marine mammal, no matter the animal's condition.

These laws, when present, are limited in their scope, typically only to emergency and initial stabilization and care. Ambulatory practitioners who encounter such cases are strongly encouraged to review the appropriate codes and regulations for their specific jurisdictions in advance to understand the limitations and protections to limit their liability.[10]

Vehicle and liability insurance

Although personal liability insurance ("malpractice") needs to be carried by the ambulatory practitioner, it is as important, if not more so, to carry appropriate vehicle insurance when practicing on an ambulatory basis. Standard homeowner's and auto owner's policies do not cover accidents, liability, damage, loss, or theft of any vehicle that is being used for business or professional purposes, nor do they cover if the vehicle is vandalized and the equipment, supplies, or other contents stolen.

Unfortunately, there is a tendency to become more litigious when one party in an accident seems to be financially solid. As a result, doctors (of any specialty), companies, and corporations are an easier target for expensive liability lawsuits and an ambulatory veterinarian must be prepared for this unfortunate eventuality. Although it is advised that a certified public accountant and a business attorney be consulted before making any decisions, it is generally safest for practitioners to operate within the scope of a personally held professional limited liability corporation or equivalent. Business insurance provides for loss and damage if scheduled, and provides appropriate coverage for accident liability. Additionally, in cases of property damage or personal injury, many insurance suppliers also provide legal counsel to defend you and their stake in the claim.

SUMMARY

Ambulatory exotic animal practice, like any veterinary practice, has specific legal issues and risks that need to be known and addressed before they become a significant issue. Many of these are the same as for any "brick-and-mortar" clinic, but others are modified or altogether unique to the mobile practice. With some basic research and consultations with legal professionals, a practitioner can dramatically reduce their liability so that they can focus on the practice of medicine and caring for their patients.

REFERENCES

1. Hemley G, editor. International wildlife trade: a CITES sourcebook. Washington, DC: Island Press, for World Wildlife Fund; 1994.
2. Available at: http://www.nmfs.noaa.gov/pr/laws/mmpa/mmpa_factsheet.pdf. Accessed December 15, 2017.
3. Available at: https://www.fisheries.noaa.gov/topic/marine-life-viewing-guidelines/guidelines-distances. Accessed January 21, 2018.
4. Stoskopf MK. Fish pharmacotherapeutics. In: Fowler ME, Miller RE, editors. Zoo and wild animal medicine: current therapy. 4th edition. Philadelphia: WB Saunders; 1999. p. 182.
5. Nolen RS. Senators unanimously approve MUMS bill. J Am Vet Med Assoc 2004; 224(8):1225–6.
6. Nolen RS. Veterinary mobility act passes congress. J Am Vet Med Assoc 2014; 245(4):358–61.
7. Available at: https://www.avma.org/Advocacy/StateAndLocal/Documents/vcpr_and_prescriptions.pdf. Accessed March 1, 2018.
8. Wilson JF. Professional liability: content, requirements, and legal implications. In: Wilson JF, Rollin BE, Garbe JAL, editors. Law and ethics of the veterinary profession. Morrisville (NC): Publishers Network; 2000. p. 155–6.
9. Scott KJ. Bailment and veterinary malpractice: doctrinal exclusivity, or not. Hastings LJ 2003;55:1009.
10. Stewart PH, Agin WS, Douglas SP. What does the law say to Good Samaritans?: a review of Good Samaritan statutes in 50 states and on US airlines. Chest 2013; 43(6):1774–83.

The Veterinary Technician in Ambulatory Exotic Animal Medicine

Erica Mede, CVT[a,b],*

KEYWORDS

- Ambulatory • Exotic • Technician • Anesthesia • Surgery • Emergency
- Diagnostics

KEY POINTS

- Equipment and inventory management includes delicate diagnostic equipment.
- Transport and safe disposal of pharmaceuticals, sharps, and legend medications is crucial.
- There are many diagnostic laboratory testing challenges.
- Client communication methods and remote second-hand observation are critical areas of discussion.
- Techniques require handling emergency situations during onsite visits.

INTRODUCTION

Veterinary technicians are exceptionally versatile by the very nature of their jobs. Technicians embarking on ambulatory medicine with their veterinarian face more challenges than are normally found in a clinic setting. It is challenging work, often requiring considerable research on species (restraint, handling, anesthetic recommendations, normal values, etc), strong time management skills, leadership, and versatility when presented with unforeseen complications and emergencies. The purpose of this article is to illuminate some of the challenges that technicians face. Veterinary technology continues to grow and expand. As it does, one area of literature will be focused on the role of veterinary technicians in the ambulatory field. At the time of this writing, however, there is little regarding technicians in exotic animal–focused ambulatory medicine written, although these authors look forward to more of it in the future.

Disclosure: The author has nothing to disclose.
[a] Exotic, Zoo, and Wildlife, Chicago Exotics Animal Hospital, 3757 W Dempster Street, Skokie, IL 60076, USA; [b] Friends of Scales Reptile Rescue, PO Box 553, Wheeling, IL 60090, USA
* 97 West Manchester Drive, Wheeling, IL 60090.
E-mail address: e.medecvt@gmail.com

Vet Clin Exot Anim 21 (2018) 563–578
https://doi.org/10.1016/j.cvex.2018.05.009
1094-9194/18/© 2018 Elsevier Inc. All rights reserved.

SCHEDULING

Scheduling ambulatory medicine appointments for exotic animals is often problematic compared with appointments at brick and mortar animal hospitals. Creating a calendar and protocol for scheduling will provide veterinary team members and clients with clear ideas of when appointments, surgeries, and follow-ups are available. One method used by this author is to review a calendar year and mark when key staff members have preplanned time off, mark the busy season(s) for your clinic, and notate any factors that will affect scheduling. This author recommends having 3 to 6 months mapped out in this manner. After 6 months, it may be difficult to reliably predict the schedule, resulting in potential mishaps including rescheduling clients. This approach is often necessary around the spring and fall when koi ponds and reproductive activity are in full swing. Department of Agriculture inspections vary by state, but are cluster scheduled by inspectors and it is useful to know when annual walk-throughs happen. Technicians should create a scheduling system with the veterinarian that includes a standardization of which day(s) of the week on-site visits can be scheduled, but also allowing for emergency examinations and follow-up appointments.

Timing

Generally, assume that an on-site visit will take twice as long as it would in the clinic for the same procedures. Travel time is factored in with external factors including traffic, rush hour, construction, and weather. A physical examination on a healthy pot-bellied pig at a home 60 miles from the clinic may take 45 minutes on-site, start to finish with sedation, examination, sample collection, and reversal. Additionally, travel time must be included. For example, a visit may take 1.5 hours of travel there, 45 minutes for the preprocedure tasks, including client discussion, and another 90 minutes back to the clinic (**Table 1**). A technician in a clinic setting may schedule a routine annual for 45 minutes in the hospital but must allow 4 hours for the same visit onsite. Ideally, scheduling of multiple visits in an area reduces time out of office and increases productivity. These "cluster appointments" are not always possible. However, with good planning, routing, and scheduling, 2 to 4 on-site visits may be the typical accommodation for a workday.

Staff Requirements

Minimally, an on-site visit will require:

- A veterinarian (preferably with a Drug Enforcement Agency [DEA] license),
- A veterinary technician (preferably proficient in laboratory procedures and anesthesia), and
- A point person at the clinic (run payments, etc).

Table 1
Comparison of appointment completion times for a pot-bellied pig examination from 60 miles away

Clinic Visit	On-Site Visit
Sedation: 15 minutes	Travel to site: 60 minutes
Physical examination: 20 minutes	Set-up and sedation: 30 minutes
Reversal and send home: 15 minutes	Physical examination: 40 minutes
Total time: 50 minutes	Reversal and pack-up: 30 minutes
	Travel to clinic: 60 minutes
	Total time: 3 hours 40 minutes

Adding more staff may seem like it will accelerate the process—after all, more hands cover more work—except with on-site visits. There are few circumstances where more than 2 staff members being out of the clinic will be beneficial to the appointment and/or conducive to an expeditious, low-stress on-site appointment. Even larger exotic animals that may be dangerous require fewer hands from the clinic. Instead, rely on the expertise of the keepers/owners at this point. If you are sure to need more people, bring them; however, always be judicious with staffing.

Location

Be aware of where on-site procedures are scheduled. If state lines are crossed, credentialed veterinary professionals will not be legal to practice medicine in the state unless licensed there. Many times, practices that are positioned close to a state line will see a mixture of in-state and out-of-state clients without problem. In ambulatory medicine, the client location is one of the top considerations in scheduling the appointment as well as later follow-up appointments.

Zoologic Facilities

Small zoologic facilities, nature centers, and serpentariums are frequent users of on-site visits (**Box 1**). Species of animals generally vary greatly at these facilities and requires prior notice for the veterinary team members to research as needed. An excellent reference for zoologic facilities to start is *Fowler's Zoo and Wild Animal Medicine* Volume 8 from Elsevier Health Sciences. A basic working knowledge for the attending veterinary team is required.

Zoologic facilities require a veterinary walk through of the exhibit animals and a review of their housing, enrichment, dietary, and sanitation protocols annually. Individual animal examinations and immunization such as rabies vaccine administration is required annually as well. In facilities housing primates and/or great apes, *Mycobacterium tuberculosis* testing will be performed, evaluated within 72 hours, and reported. Clinicians may opt to evaluate results via e-mail or other electronic imaging. This process runs the risk of a false reading and a challenge that technicians should discuss with their veterinarians before scheduling the visit if possible.

Technicians may be required to use various capture methods including dart guns, nets, ropes, and various pole length apparatuses. Generally, facility staff are versed in these methods of restraint and will offer valuable assistance in the use of different equipment.

Private Collections

The public often has unique and varied personal collections of animals in their homes. Some are breeders, some are collectors of a certain genus, and some are people that enjoy unique pets (**Box 2**). Personal ponds are a popular addition to most homes in

---

Box 1
Typical reasons for zoologic facility on-site visits

- Annual examinations
- Acute problems (trauma, emergency, bacteriosis, etc)
- Chronic problems (geriatrics, disease management, etc)
- Inspections
- Reproductive reasons (birthing, complications, etc)

Box 2
Typical reasons for private sector client on-site visits

- Ponds
- Large aquarium fish (including sharks)
- Aggressive and/or dangerous animals (crocodilians, felids, venomous reptiles, etc)
- Inability to safely transport the animal to the clinic
- Large animals (pot-bellied pigs, crocodilians, exotic hoof stock, etc)
- Large reptile collections
- Large and/or highly varied menagerie
- Distance from the clinic
- Delicate species (bats, large invertebrate collection, etc)

---

suburban and semirural areas and are often stocked with ornamental fish. Exotic animals are easily made available to the clients through auctions and breeders in person and, more frequently, online. The state, county, and/or township your client lives in is an important factor. Another consideration is space to work. When scheduling appointments with clients in the private sector, inform them that the animal will need to be contained/captured before arrival and a clear work place will be necessary to expedite the appointment.

Surgical Calls

Surgical procedures on-site are more commonly minor in nature with minimal invasiveness but can extend to emergency procedures of all forms. The choice to perform field surgery depends on the practice and regulations of the state in which you are practicing medicine. Surgical interventions on-site will generally consume significantly more time than normally allotted in the clinic. A suitable surgical area will need to be created that ensures the veterinarian has the appropriate tools, lighting, anesthesia, and other necessary surgical supplies easily accessible.

US Department of Agriculture Animal and Plant Health Inspection Service Licensed Facilities

US Department of Agriculture Plant Health Inspection Service Plant Health Inspection Service licensed facilities (**Box 3**) are a little more difficult to schedule. The US

Box 3
US Department of Agriculture Plant Health Inspection Service classifications

Class A: Breeders and dealers who sell animals that are bred and raised in a closed colony

Class B: Dealers that purchase and/or resell warm-blooded animals

Class C: Exhibitors with warm-blooded animal on display that perform for the public or in educational presentations

Data from United States Department of Agriculture: Animal and Plant Health Inspection Service (USDA/APHIS). Regulated Businesses (Licensing and Registration.) Available at: https://www.aphis.usda.gov/aphis/ourfocus/animalwelfare/ct_awa_regulated_businesses. Accessed February 4, 2018.

Department of Agriculture requires an annual on-site inspection and review of facility protocols by a veterinarian. Often, they will try to have the mandatory annual examinations performed at the same time, as well as any vaccinations required. Site inspections without physical examinations will take less time than site inspections with examinations included, depending on the size of the facility, the species maintained, the volume of animals, and the scope of the visit (**Box 4**).

EQUIPMENT

Technicians in the clinic have all the necessary tools and pharmaceuticals present on-site that they need to process and expedite appointments. On-site, technicians must anticipate the needs of their veterinarian before leaving the hospital. When packing equipment, consider bringing extra frequently used items such as gauze (**Box 5**). Consider keeping items from ambulatory medicine separate from the general animal hospital supplies to ensure you always have necessary items and contamination is minimized.

Mobile Technology

Smart phones are the talk of most veterinary management social sites both in a positive light and negative light.[1] During on-site visits, smart phones and tablet computers are useful for the applications that can be downloaded and the variety of products that can be purchased for phones as well. Multiport charging apparatuses for vehicles as well as emergency power sources are well worth considering when working out of the office. With these systems always changing, it is beyond the scope of this article to completely discuss applications and equipment that can are available.

An electronic reader application on the smart phone is invaluable for accessing reference material while on a site visit. Applications such as Zoetis Fluid Calculator can be used on site and some drug calculators can be modified for clinician preferences. The following references should be considered as useful in ambulatory exotic animal medicine:

- *Fowler's Zoo and Wildlife* (multiple editions),
- *Plumb's Veterinary Drug Handbook,*
- *Carpenter's Exotic Animal Formulary,*
- Laboratory references, and
- Anesthetic references.

Box 4
Exceptions to US Department of Agriculture Plant Health Inspection Service licensing

- Retail pet stores

- Breeders with 4 or fewer breeding female dogs, cats, and/or small exotic or wild mammals

- Dealers who sell fewer than 25 dogs or cats a year to research facilities

- Dealers who purchase and sell animals for food or fiber

- Any person who purchases animals solely for their personal enjoyment

Data from United States Department of Agriculture: Animal and Plant Health Inspection Service (USDA/APHIS). Regulated Businesses (Licensing and Registration). Available at: https://www.aphis.usda.gov/aphis/ourfocus/animalwelfare/ct_awa_regulated_businesses. Accessed February 4, 2018.

Box 5
Pharmaceuticals for cardiopulmonary resuscitation crash kits

- Norepinephrine or epinephrine
- Dopamine
- Atropine
- Glycopyrrolate
- Furosemide
- Benzodiazepines
- Fluids for fluid therapy
- Corticosteroids
- Lidocaine

Applications include medical record notes such as Evernote or OneNote, driving directions through Google Maps, financial applications such as QuickBooks, and ease of keeping photographic records of patient progress through applications such as OneDrive, Picasso, and other storage options that allow for categorizing. Cloud-based digital services allow for team members onsite and at the clinic access to the same information.[2]

The "Go Box"

Unless you have an ambulatory vehicle where you can keep all necessary equipment and pharmaceuticals stocked and available, you will need a dedicated "Go Box." This box should be easy to move, preferably on wheels and water resistant. Go Boxes must be easy to disinfect and water resistant. Tool boxes with all terrain wheels are strongly recommended for outdoor endeavors.

Often, multiple transport containers are used based on the needs of the appointment. For instance, a general medical examination box may contain laboratory diagnostics, pharmaceuticals, paper work, and generalized medical supplies (**Box 6**). A surgical medical box should be maintained separately containing sterile items, a lock box that meets DEA standards for controlled pharmaceuticals, and necessary equipment. DEA regulations regarding legend drugs can be found on the DEA's resources under Part 1301 of the Code of Federal Regulations.[3]

A thorough inventory system must be in place to prevent leaving behind supplies. An inventory should be performed before leaving the clinic and after the appointment before returning to the clinic. This author uses a printed out check list that is customized for each visit. The travel sheet has the date of the visit, client information, list of supplies brought, and check boxes for items brought to the visit, items that are returning to the clinic, and one for item dispensed to owners. Sharps, such as needles, are accounted for and the number noted on the travel sheet. Used sharps must be placed in a regulation biohazard container designated for the use of disposal of sharps as described by Occupational Safety & Health Administration Blood Borne Pathogen Standards.[4]

Pharmaceuticals

Before scheduling on-site visits, a system to address pharmaceutical handling and dispensing is necessary. Prescriptions that need to be submitted to a compounding

---

Box 6
General medical supplies and pharmaceuticals for house calls

General supplies

- Nonlatex examination gloves
- Tongue depressors
- Cotton-tipped applicators (sterile and unsterile)
- Hands-free lighting
- Gauze (sterile and unsterile)
- Clipboard with examination forms, necessary forms, etc
- Nail clippers
- Dremmel with appropriate grooming bits
- Grooming scissors
- Basic bandage material
- Syringes and needles
- Suture packs
- Dental rasps as needed

Pharmaceuticals

- Appropriate antibiotics
- Eye medications
- Ear cleanser
- Benzodiazepine injectables
- Nonsteroidal antiinflammatory drugs
- Sedatives
- Wound cleanser

---

pharmacy can be created on-site through a phone call directly to the pharmacy or at the clinic. Most clients are happy to allow you to use their WiFi, if not, many cell phones can be turned into mobile hotspots. Prescriptions filled on site are required to adhere to state and federal dispensing regulations and will require appropriate labeling.

Controlled substances and anesthetics should be transported in a locked container that can withstand the motion and risks of transport. A controlled substance log must be maintained for the use of ambulatory medications. A separate set of controlled substance drugs can be kept for ambulatory medicine and maintained as described by the DEA.[3] A separate set of controlled substances allows for exact record keeping of use on-site and prevents interrupting hospital function back at the clinic if it is still open. The technician's greatest challenge with on-site visits, other than keeping veterinarians on time, is maintaining inventory of pharmaceuticals.

Along with the pharmaceuticals, appropriate paraphernalia must be brought to the site. These include:

- Dispensing bottles,
- Appropriate warning labels, and
- Administration devices (oral syringes, flush syringes, injectables, etc).

Keeping a formulary and/or pharmaceutical reference on your smart phone is advised unless a copy is available.

Surgical Equipment

Surgical procedures may be indicated during on-site visits. It is recommended, unless you have the facilities onsite, to perform invasive surgeries in the hospital. Surgical equipment should be packed in a way that minimizes potential contamination and extra supplies must always be on hand.

Anesthesia machines can be transported; however, consider the state regulations for transporting halogenated ethers, oxygen, carbon dioxide, and/or nitrous oxide. Vehicles may be required to note what is being carried. The list of anesthesia paraphernalia is listed in **Box 7** is illustrative, not exhaustive.

This is not taking into consideration aquatic or pond calls. Anticipate to the best of your ability the veterinarian's needs, the condition being addressed, and the species to be examined, and pack accordingly. The author recommends using a surgical checklist as well. This list differs from an inventory list and will be tailored to the upcoming appointment. Resuscitation devices are ideal for maintaining patients after anesthesia has finished until full recovery with positive pressure ventilation. This method is particularly useful in reptiles, ideally with automatic ventilators[5] (**Box 8**).

Blankets, towels, and portable thermoregulatory devices need to be brought with. Active warming devices are recommended over passive devices. Active warming systems can be used to create tailored temperatures, are controllable, and offer consistency to prevent hypothermia. Passive warming systems such as hot water bottles and heat disks are uncontrollable and will start to leach heat from the patient once the patient is warmer than the heating element.[6]

Box 7
Suggested anesthesia paraphernalia

- Halogenated ether vaporizer
- Oxygen tank (preferably on a wheeled cart)
- Scuba tank (excellent for providing ventilation to large animals including crocodilians)
- Extra isoflurane/halothane/sevoflurane
- Nitrous oxide canister
- Carbon dioxide canister
- F-Air containers (multiple for longer procedures or large animals)
- Face masks
- Endotracheal tubes and/or supraglottic air way devices
- Laryngoscopes with multiple blades and/or rigid endoscope
- Rebreathing and nonrebreathing systems (preferably 2 in case an infectious animal is examined)
- Multiple appropriately sized reservoir bags (multiple sizes are suggested)
- Anesthetic induction chambers
- Eye lubricant
- Human resuscitation devices such as AMBU bags

Box 8
Equipment to consider bringing on house calls

- A cart or dolly with good wheels capable of holding greater than 250 lbs
- Scale
- Buckets (especially for aquatic appointments)
- Handling equipment (snake hooks, snake tubes, catch poles, towels, gloves, etc)
- Human first aid kit
- Cleansing solutions to disinfect equipment
- Towels (more than you think)
- Garbage bags
- Portable lighting
- Rope, twine, and zip-ties
- Plastic sheeting (protect floors, offer work spaces, etc)
- Portable folding table

Many devices can perform multiple tasks, reducing the amount of equipment that needs to be brought on a visit (**Box 9**). It remains the gold standard to have multiple devices and methods of life support available for safeguarding the patient. It may prevent an emergency if there is mechanical failure. Smaller multipurpose units such as the Sentier Vetcorder (Sentier, Brookfield, WI) are easy to transport, reliable, and affordable for most veterinary practices.

Diagnostic Considerations

Scheduling appointments for on-site calls is difficult, especially when it comes to laboratory testing. A technician in the clinic has equipment to expedite their laboratory specimen evaluation. As a mobile technician in the field, it may not be possible due to the availability of portable laboratory equipment. Although microscopes are easily transported to sites and a skilled technician can perform cytology, fecal analysis, urinalysis, and blood smears evaluations immediately on-site, other techniques may require returning samples to the stationary clinic or submission to a reference

---

Box 9
Other monitoring devices to bring

- Electrocardiograph
- Pulse oximeter
- Thermometer
- Blood pressure monitors
- Stethoscope
- SPO_2 monitor
- End-tidal CO_2 monitor
- Doppler ultrasound monitor

---

laboratory. In these cases, it is critical for the technician to be well-versed in the proper collection, processing, storage, and transport of these samples for an accurate and reliable analysis.

Portable radiographic and ultrasonography units are available and have the benefit of offering immediate information. Imaging units are delicate, and their size may make vehicle accommodations difficult, but will offer valuable diagnostics. Veterinary technicians will need to be versed in maintenance, trouble shooting, and use of equipment brought on-site.

LABORATORY
Sample Collection

Sample collection even in the clinic can be difficult in exotic species for the veterinary technician. On-site visits pose a different set of challenges including:

- Poor lighting,
- Restraint (potential lack of available and/or appropriately trained assistance),
- Limited supplies (especially in multiple examination visits),
- Inquisitive owners,
- Patients who are difficult to control in their home environment, and
- Biohazard spill potential.

The most important key to success for the technician is flexibility and resourcefulness. The comfort and safety of the patient and people are paramount. The veterinary technician attending on-site calls needs to be well-versed in venipuncture to expedite procedures and diagnostics. A thorough working understanding of proper restraint techniques is required to assist the veterinarian on-site and/or offer crash courses to owners, assistants, and other caretakers. Technicians should be proficient in aseptic techniques to avoid contamination of the sample and the necessity to repeat the testing.

On-Site Evaluation

Travel microscopes are integral assets for the ambulatory visit. The ability to expeditiously evaluate diagnostic samples on-site is invaluable. Unfortunately, if a diagnostic quality microscope is not brought with you, diagnostics will be delayed further. It may be tempting to bring a lesser microscope, but you will end up working twice as hard having to reevaluate samples (**Box 10**).

Stains such as gram stain sets, and rapid differential stain kits are easy to transport and add value to your diagnostics. The ability to evaluate a patient's cytologic sample can prevent a delay in diagnosis and treatment. Transportation of samples can cause artifacts and delay diagnosis. A veterinary technician evaluating a cytologic sample allows the veterinarian the chance to continue with the rest of the appointment. Timing and multitasking are traits both admirable in the clinic and essential on-site regarding diagnostic testing.

Transportation

Samples that are collected and cannot be evaluated immediately or will be submitted for further testing need to be transported in a way that does not negatively affect the sample integrity. Considerations include:

- Insulated container,
- Icepacks and/or cooling packs (not dry ice), and
- Padding.

Box 10
Common samples collected on-site

- Urinalysis and culture
- Blood for culture, complete blood count, serum chemistry, PCR, ELISA, snap tests, platelet evaluation, and blood typing, etc
- Cytology for FNA evaluation, skin scrapes, gill clips, PCR, ELISA, cultures, special stain evaluations, etc
- Feces for parasite analysis, fecal floatation, stain evaluation, culture, PCR, ELISA, etc
- Swabs from cloacas, choanas, ears, noses, etc
- Tracheal washes
- Gastric washes
- Celiocentesis
- Tear production tests
- Heavy metal testing
- Milk for cultures, etc

Abbreviations: ELISA, enzyme-linked immunosorbent assay; FNA, fine needle aspiration; PCR, polymerase chain reaction.

A technician should put extra care into the packing and shipping of samples, especially during extreme weather such as excessive heat. For this reason, icepacks are used to prevent the sample from warming with the added benefit of preventing iatrogenic damage owing to freezing.

Medical Biowaste

Samples contaminated with potential infectious agents should be treated as biohazardous material and transported in a double barrier manner. Barrier material should be nonporous and impermeable. Discarded samples and collection devices should be placed in sharps containers and/or red biohazard bags for proper disposal. Biomedical waste should be clearly marked and, when possible, transported separately. Avoid the temptation to use 1 biomedical/biohazard bag for all house calls on a day. This option may seem fiscally advantageous, especially when based on weight, but it can lead to the spreading of pathogens and nosocomial infections. Infectious waste, pharmaceuticals, and sharps should be removed with the technician during departure for appropriate biohazard disposal.

It is advisable for the technician to research the state Department of Natural Resources regulations to avoid violations.

The following need to be handled properly and are often overlooked on ambulatory calls:

- Sharps (needles, syringes, scalpels, etc),
- Animal waste (carcasses, biological waste, contaminated materials, etc), and
- Hazardous waste (pharmaceutical waste).

The Department of Transportation requires you to[7]:

- Clearly label all hazardous material,
- Store waste in rigid containers (leak proof, tamper proof, spill proof, and puncture resistant),

- Ability to provide cradle to grave manifestations (ie, where it was created to where it was destroyed and what it was), and
- Permits are required when there is more than 50 pounds of waste.

There are several options for disposal with mail-back options being an option as well.

CLIENT COMMUNICATIONS

Communications with the client must be recorded. There are phone applications available that track the amount of time spent on a phone call with clients. E-mail is an easy way to convey information to clients as well as convenient for the busy technician. E-mails are a staple for continuity as well as detailed notes regarding:

- Discussion topic,
- Owner concerns/questions,
- Recommendations made,
- Any changes to treatment plan or therapies (and who authorized them), and
- Changes to the diagnosis and/or prognosis.

Accurate record keeping should be a primary goal of the veterinary team. As discussed, note taking on cloud-based applications such as Evernote and OneNote can be used for medical notes. Veterinary software such as Idexx provides mobile options through installation on tablets and laptops that can be brought on-site.

E-mail offers an advantage to ambulatory practices allowing veterinary staff to view photographs of the patient as well as video from the client directly. E-mail is beneficial for clients a great distance from the clinic. Charting progress is easier with constant communication being made available to you and the client. However, challenges can arise including confidentiality, accountability, and a potential drain of resources such as time. Technicians and practitioners operating e-mail must outline what they will and will not discuss over e-mails as well as guidelines for answering e-mails. For instance, do you only respond to e-mails during work hours or can clients contact you whenever they wish? Who will respond to e-mails and in what time frame? This author's clinic uses e-mail and the guidelines set in the clinic prohibit diagnosis over e-mail and appointment scheduling. An automated response can be sent to all e-mails that states your clinic's guidelines such as, "Thank you for contacting us. We will respond as soon as we are able during scheduled work hours, which are Monday through Friday from 8 AM to 6 PM and Saturday from 8 AM to 2 PM If this is regarding an emergency or to make an appointment, please call us at 555-555-5555."

When patients are not presented to the clinic physically for a follow-up evaluation, it can be difficult to assess progress. Photographs and videos are not meant to replace examinations, but are meant as an adjunct.

POND FISH CONSIDERATIONS

Pond side calls are one of the more labor-intensive calls a technician can attend. They often require wading into ponds or at the very least working long nets to capture fish, generally koi, patients. Technicians must safely and expeditiously setup the mobile clinic in often less than ideal conditions, especially where the weather is concerned. Considerations when scouting an appropriate location for on-site visits include:

- Shade,
- Lighting,

- Protection from the elements, and
- Place to setup a table for supplies and work.

Ideally, owners will already have the fish in question segregated from the rest of the pond. Unfortunately, it does not always occur this way. When a fish must be retrieved, often it is up to the technician to capture the fish, preferably with the netting used normally by the owner to prevent cross-contamination of systems (and having to transport wet cargo). It is advisable to bring hip-high waders and a net in case you are required to use your own equipment. Nonslip rubberized mats add additional safety to a potentially slick work area if multiple trips are needed and/or the fish patient is "splashy."

Once the patient is captured, it is the technician's duty to restrain the fish in a way that allows for optimal safety, minimal restraint time, and, most important, in a way that will not offend the owner. Bus boy trays or concrete mixing trays can be used for a fish examination area. These trays are inexpensive, versatile, and easily disinfected between uses. Bubble wrap is another option to prevent trauma to the patient with the added benefit of offering comfort to the owner that their pet is being cared for delicately.

An example of a typical start to a pond call includes:

- Veterinarian talks with the client while setup occurs,
- Technician captures fish, and
- Fish is evaluated briefly and often sedated soon after weighing to reduce stress.

It is important that samples are collected quickly and as much detail as can be reasonably recorded reported for accuracy of further testing, especially when multiple fish are being collected from.

Disposal of water containing tricaine methanesulfonate (MS-222) must be done safely. It is highly recommended to check with local governing and waste authorities to determine the legal and appropriate methods of disposal within that jurisdiction.

Microscopes, and subsequently the extension cords, are essential for effective pond calls. Using water-resistant materials or sleeves to protect electrical cords/equipment and other sealing methods is encouraged to prevent tripping hazards as well as minimize electrical problems. Many parasites can be diagnosed quickly, and appropriate treatments started. A sample of water can be evaluated:

- Microscopically,
- For water quality (kits that require mixing or test strips), and
- For specific gravity.

A pearl of wisdom when it comes to cytologic evaluation of gill clips, skin scrapes, and mucus smears is to use the water the fish naturally lives in rather than sterile saline.[8]

EMERGENCY SITUATIONS

Emergency medical situations are part of any ambulatory exotic animal practice (**Box 11**). In the veterinary clinic, they can be addressed immediately with all available equipment, personnel, pharmaceuticals, and privacy. On-site, privacy is not always a luxury afforded to the veterinary staff nor all the necessary equipment and/or pharmaceuticals. Emergency situations encountered on site visits include:

- Iatrogenic trauma during capture/restraint,
- Capture cardiomyopathy,

Box 11
Equipment to consider bringing on house calls for laboratory diagnostics

- Microscope
- Microscope slides and cover slips
- Mineral oil
- Immersion oil
- Fecal float medium
- Portable small centrifuge
- Culture and sensitivity collection materials
- PCR or virology collection materials
- Hematocrit tubes with PCV reader
- Urinalysis stain
- Urinalysis dip sticks
- Cytologic stain kits
- Lighter or other flame source
- Otoscope
- Ophthalmoscope

Abbreviations: PCR, polymerase chain reaction; PCV, packed cell value.

- Anesthetic emergencies,
- Seizures,
- Various other issues secondary to a disease or injury process, and
- Vaccine reactions.

This list is illustrative, but gives an idea of situations that may arise regarding the patient. Other nonmedical situations that can become critical that the technician must take into consideration include:

- Vehicular issues transporting a patient back to the clinic,
- Personnel injury while caring for or restraining the patient, and
- Weather-related (storms, snow drifts, tornados, etc) conditions that prolong travel and care of the patient.

Ambulatory technicians must be versatile and quickly able to adapt to a changing, potentially volatile, situation in a manner that does not raise further alarm for the owner or veterinarian. Clear communication with the veterinarian on-site and a scenario-based discussion before appointments is encouraged. This author uses the car rides to sites with her veterinarian to dialogue desired outcomes, potential issues that may arise, and how the situation and client should be handled at the time. As with all scenario-based dialogue, actual outcomes will vary. The desired cohesive unification and forethought regarding common scenarios, however, will be appreciated not only by those in attendance, but by the client and patient as well. To quote Benjamin Franklin's wisdom, "an ounce of prevention is worth a pound of cure."

Cardiopulmonary Resuscitation On-Site

A mobile crash kit should accompany every on-site visit. Ideally, it will not differ too greatly from what the technician and veterinarian are accustomed to at the hospital (**Box 12**). As with all lists in this article, it is illustrative and not exhaustive. Crash kits should be tailored to the appointment to the best of your ability. House calls have the additional challenge when it comes to emergency medicine of limited space to pack supplies. Opting for a smaller handheld, multiparameter measuring unit such as the Vetcorder will save space with the ability to provide 2-lead electrocardiography, pulse oximetry, and temperature readings. Pharmaceuticals include various cardiac support agents, sedatives, and ventilatory support drugs.[9]

Handling Death During Visits

Unfortunately, death does occur on ambulatory calls; whether they are the reason for the call determines the client's response. Acute death owing to pharmaceutical reactions, anesthesia, or complications during restraint or a procedure are often handled differently by the owner than if the pet perished after illness, injury, or request for euthanasia.

At a veterinary hospital, there is a degree of separation from the client and the incident. This is not always the case on house calls, which can lead to emotionally charged situations. For this reason, it is always best to be transparent with owners that there is always a chance of sudden and unexpected terminal complications, when appropriate. Reviewing protocols with the veterinarian before an appointment, even in the car ride to the site, is advised to reduce the burden to both the owner and the veterinary team.

Deceased animals must be transported as biohazard waste.[10] The method of preparing a body for transportation can seem callous, especially regarding placing the deceased in an approved container that may require the deceased to be folded/contorted. For this reason, it is best to cover the body and request the owner leave before packing the patient up. It is of the utmost importance that the body is treated carefully and with respect. Check with the state practiced in on any regulations regarding disposal of cadavers if the client requests the patient be left. If the cadaver is to be

---

Box 12
A well-stocked crash kit includes

- Pharmaceuticals
- Delivery systems including intravenous access
- Sterile saline flushes (heparinized and nonheparinized)
- Tourniquets
- Monitoring equipment
- Pen light or other small light source
- Temperature regulating devices (ice packs, heat pads, etc)
- Eye lubricant
- Air way devices (air sac cannulas, tracheostomy tubes, endotracheal tubes, etc)
- Suction devices
- Pediatric and adult-human ventilators and/or bag valve masks
- Oxygen canister with regulator
- Scuba tank with regulator

left behind for the owner to handle on their own, it should be done, again, in a respectful manner preferably covered to convey sympathies.

SUMMARY

Veterinary technicians in ambulatory services will face unique challenges that mirror those found in the clinic but vary with difficulty to overcome owing to ambulatory medicine being complicated to predict at times. Versatility, knowledge of species and disease processes, and an ability to multitask are important skills to hone to succeed. As the field of veterinary medicine expands and continues to change, this author hopes that veterinary technology will continue to grow and a specialty in ambulatory medicine will become a pursuable career option.

REFERENCES

1. Frankel C. Be smart about using smartphones in practice. 2015. Available at: https://www.veterinaryteambrief.com/article/be-smart-about-using-smartphones-practice. Accessed February 4, 2018.
2. Jergler D. Embrace the world of veterinary apps. 2014. Available at: https://www.veterinarypracticenews.com/embrace-the-world-of-veterinary-apps/. Accessed February 4, 2018.
3. US Drug Enforcement Administration (DEA). N.D. Title 21 code of federal regulations. Available at: https://www.deadiversion.usdoj.gov/21cfr/cfr/2101cfrt.htm. Accessed February 4, 2018.
4. US Department of Labor Occupation Safety and Health Administration (OSHA), 2015. Disposal of contaminated needles and blood holders used for phlebotomy. Available at: https://www.osha.gov/dts/shib/shib101503.html. Accessed February 4, 2018.
5. Spielvogel C, King L, Cavin JM, et al. Use of positive pressure ventilation in cold-stunned sea turtles: 29 cases (2008-2014). J Herpetol Med Surg 2017;27(1–2): 48–57.
6. Byers CG. Cold critters: understanding hypothermia. 2012. Available at: http://veterinarymedicine.dvm360.com/cold-critters-understanding-hypothermia. Accessed February 4, 2018.
7. Federal Motor Carrier Safety Administration, 2014. How to comply with federal hazardous materials regulations. Accessed February 4, 2018.
8. Francis-Floyd R. Fish. In: Kahn CM, editor. The Merck veterinary manual. 9th edition. Whitehouse Station (NJ): Merck & Co., Inc; 2005. p. 1479–516.
9. Kirby R. Evaluation and initial treatment of the emergency patient. In: Kahn C, editor. The Merck's veterinary manual. 9th edition. Whitestation (NJ): Merck & Co; 2005. p. 1394–9.
10. Meri Inc, ND. Three tips for compliant veterinary medical waste disposal. Available at: https://www.meriinc.com/three-tips-for-compliant-veterinary-medical-waste-disposal/. Accessed December 19, 2017.

Sample Collection

Kendal E. Harr, DVM, MS, DACVP

KEYWORDS

- Quality management • American Society for Veterinary Clinical Pathology
- Lymphodilution • Jugular vein

KEY POINTS

- Deviation from recommended protocols can adversely affect test results resulting in incorrect diagnoses.
- Quality management of samples must start in the patient, extend through sampling itself, include appropriate short transport and then be correctly accessioned at the referral laboratory or in-house station to ensure accurate diagnosis of disease.
- Information concerning sample requirements, proper collection, handling, and delivery or shipping procedures for any assay performed at a referral laboratory should be available to the veterinarian electronically, in written materials.
- These materials should be maintained in the clinic in a manner easily accessible to staff.
- Specimens should be handled carefully and transported to the laboratory in a timely manner under conditions appropriate for the type of sample and its stability.
- Contact manufacturers for specific details that are available digitally or in writing.

REQUIRED SAMPLE COLLECTION MANUAL AND PERSONNEL

Samples should be collected according to standard practices that are detailed herein. Deviation from recommended protocols can adversely affect test results. Information concerning sample requirements, proper collection, handling, and delivery or shipping procedures for any assay performed at a referral laboratory should be available to the veterinarian electronically, in written materials (such as a laboratory services manual, special information sheets, etc), and should be maintained in the clinic in a manner easily accessible to staff at all times. According to American Society for Veterinary Clinical Pathology guidelines,[1] detailed sample collection protocols should be available from your referral laboratory and you can simply call to receive the manual. If you are running these analysis in your clinic, you have taken on the responsibility of collecting and organizing all of this information. Instrument manufacturer's package inserts have detailed descriptions of appropriate samples, including collection tubes and handling conditions. The specimens should be handled carefully and transported to the laboratory in a timely manner under conditions appropriate for the type of sample and its stability. Contact manufacturers for specific details, which are available

Disclosure: The author has nothing to disclose.
URIKA, LLC, 8712, 53rd Pl W, Mukilteo, WA 98275, USA
E-mail address: drharr@urikapathology.com

Vet Clin Exot Anim 21 (2018) 579–592
https://doi.org/10.1016/j.cvex.2018.05.008
1094-9194/18/© 2018 Elsevier Inc. All rights reserved.

digitally or in writing. A quality assurance plan at the laboratory chosen is mandatory under ASVCP guidelines.

Laboratory and veterinary clinic personnel should have specific training in sampling, specimen handling, and sample preparation for exotic species contained in this article. Training should include basic prevention of bacterial contamination as well as information on zoonotic diseases including *Chlamydia*, West Nile Virus, Salmonella, avian influenza, Giardia, and any other diseases likely to be encountered in the practice. Documentation of training, continuing education, and periodic proficiency assessment should be done annually at the direction of the clinic and/or laboratory director.[2]

BLOOD COLLECTION

The smallest needle size appropriate to the species and sample volume should be used, which is most commonly a 22- to 25-G needle in medium to small species. Smaller gauges should not be used because shear forces will result in increased cell lysis and poor sample quality. Samples with moderate to severe hemolysis should be flagged or rejected by your laboratory.[1] Larger gauges may be required in larger reptiles to penetrate the scaled dermis and may make blood collection faster. Consider using a stylet to prevent dermal and tissue plugs in the blood sample, which can stimulate clotting.

Calculate the maximum safe blood volume before collection. Reptilian total blood volume is approximately 5% to 8% of bodyweight. In a healthy normovolemic animal, 10% of the blood volume can be collected safely, that is, 0.5% to 0.8% of body weight (in grams). Hence, the phlebotomist can collect 0.8 mL blood from a 100-g gecko safely. Collect blood samples as soon as possible after the animal is restrained or anesthetized to minimize the effects of restraint or sedation on plasma biochemical and hematologic values.

When sampling reptiles (poikilotherms), it is important to maintain their temperature before, during, and after sampling. To accurately assess blood values, the clinician must have good temperature data from exactly where the animal is residing in their enclosure. It does not matter what the temperature is under the lamp if that is not where the animal stays in the enclosure. Lower temperatures result in lower cell counts and lower enzymatic activity in the animal.[3–6] The clinician must expect that, if animals have been chronically housed in a suboptimal temperature either by owners or in the clinic, values may be falsely lowered. When the poikilotherm is then rechecked, having been housed in the thermoneutral zone, values will increase potentially then indicating inflammation. However, the animal seems to be better clinically. This finding is to be expected and is an indication to continue therapy because the animal is still mounting a response to the likely chronic infection. It is not an indication that there is a problem with therapy. Hence, the herpetology-savvy clinician must have a good understanding of the animal's environment, including temperature, to interpret diagnostic blood data.

The clinician must also have information about recent meal consumption in addition to temperature data. A good example is the postprandial snake, which can seem to have mild azotemia and possible renal disease when the reality is that it is just well fed. It is best to ensure fasting samples in reptiles to avoid confusion. Another renal disease mimic is, of course, oviparity. Accurate identification of sex may be a problem in some species, but this information is worthwhile to pursue so that this partitioning factor is known.

Lymphodilution occurs more commonly in reptiles than in other orders of animals. Many vessels used for blood collection in reptiles are in close approximation to lymph vessels.[7] Normal lymph contains small, well-differentiated lymphocytes and variable quantities of protein and lipid, depending on location. A lymph-draining, inflamed region may be very different and reflects the immune cell population that it is draining from tissues. Because lymph is dissimilar to blood, excessive contamination may affect hematologic and biochemical values (ie, decreased hematocrit, total protein, potassium, and chloride). The heart and jugular veins seem to be the sites least likely to be contaminated by lymph.

In turtles, blood collection sites include the jugular vein, supravertebral (subcarapacial) vein, brachial vein, femoral vein, and coccygeal veins. In lizards, blood may be collected from the jugular vein, ventral coccygeal vein (tail vein) (**Fig. 1**), brachial vein, and ventral abdominal vein. Use of either cardiac puncture or toenail clips in lizards and turtles is not recommended owing to sample quality, safety, and ethical issues. In snakes, common blood collection sites include the ventral coccygeal vein, heart, and vertebral sinus. Palatine veins are not recommended owing to danger to the phlebotomist. Death has been caused by venipuncture at both the vertebral sinus and the occipital sinus, and so these sites should be used as a last resort only after training and they are, therefore, not described herein.

The largest bore vein accessible in the animal should be chosen because it is most likely to provide a high-quality sample. The jugular vein, as a general rule, is recommended because blood samples from this site typically have less cell lysis and fewer artifacts (**Fig. 2**). This site is commonly used in green iguanas, where it has been described as a blind stick midway between the ear and the point of the shoulder. In a veterinary clinic, use of the jugular vein may be challenging in other lizards due to the highly variable anatomic location between squamate species, combined with the lack of a raised vein. Ultrasound-guided venipuncture may be possible if Doppler ultrasound examination is available. In chelonia, the external jugular veins are very superficial and are located on the lateral neck. They are more dorsal than those of mammals and lie at the level of the auricular scale. An assistant or the venipuncturist gently extends the head and neck for appropriate exposure of the jugular vein. This procedure may only be possible in very ill or anesthetized animals. Anesthesia is your friend. Avoid spinal trauma due to overzealous restrain at all costs. Applying pressure at the thoracic inlet distends the vessel to facilitate visualization. A Q-tip is useful for this purpose because it does not impair visualization of the vessel. If the animal is anesthetized and intubated, positive pressure ventilation will also dilate the jugular vein. Turning the animal into a lateral position and tilting the neck may also be helpful. Large

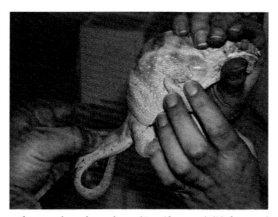

Fig. 1. Phlebotomy of a panther chameleon (*Furcifer pardalis*) from a lateral approach to the ventral caudal vein. (*Courtesy of* Adolf Maas, DVM, Bothell, WA.)

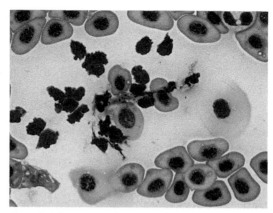

Fig. 2. Cell lysis in a bearded dragon. Small needle gauges, pushing blood back through the-needle, or any excessive vacuum or pressure from the syringe or slides can cause cells to lyse, decreasing the accuracy and validity of quantitative results. (*Modified* Wrights stain at 500× magnification)

Galapagos and Aldabra tortoises may extend their head and necks in response to neck rubbing or being hosed with water.[8]

The ventral coccygeal vein or tail vein is the most accessible blood collection site, but samples may contain small clots, bone fragments, and other debris. The vessel lies along the midventral aspect of the vertebral bodies, partly protected by the ventral spinous processes. The needle should be of sufficient length to reach the vertebral body and of an appropriate diameter relative to the vessel. For a medium lizard and snake, a 1.0- to 1.5-inch × 22- to 25-G needle attached to a 3-mL syringe can be used. A butterfly catheter attached to a syringe may also be useful. The vessel is usually approached from the ventral midline, but may also be approached laterally. The lizard is placed in either dorsal or sternal recumbency, which is preferred for large lizards that are difficult to restrain. Holding the animal vertically with the tail down will aid in gravity-assisted blood collection, as will extending the tail toward the ground from a table or open kennel. The needle is inserted in the midline and advanced until the vertebral body is contacted. The needle may be either inserted perpendicular to the ventral surface of the vertebral body or at a 45° angle to the vertebrae, to facilitate passage between the ventral spinous processes. Avoid the cloaca as well as the hemipenes in males. Once the vertebral body is contacted, a negative pressure is applied to the syringe and the needle slowly retracted until blood flow occurs. If blood does not flow, the needle position is reassessed and adjusted. Rattlesnakes that possess active muscular tails seem to have large ventral coccygeal vessels. However, even large snakes of other species may have relatively small coccygeal vessels, making blood collection difficult. The dorsal coccygeal vein is accessed most easily in giant tortoises and snapping turtles. It is located in the dorsal midline above the vertebrae. Large tortoises are gently turned on their back, causing them to curl their tails over to allow access to the dorsal midline surface. The skin must be cleaned thoroughly because of the often-heavy fecal contamination of this area. The sample taker should also be alert to kicks from these animals. This vessel extends under the shell and can sometimes be accessed by placing the needle in the midline and directing anteriorly under the posterior edge of the carapace.

The ventral abdominal vein may be accessed in the midline of the caudal abdomen immediately under the skin. The abdomens of geckos and other small lizards may be transilluminated to visualize the ventral abdominal vein, as well as the heart and other organs. Although this is an option for venous access, it is not recommended as a standard site due to potential complications, such uncontrolled hemorrhage if lacerated or abdominal contamination with intestinal contents if the underlying bowel is penetrated.

Cardiac puncture for diagnostic blood collection is only recommended in snakes and care must be taken to avoid laceration in active animals. The position of the snake heart varies between species. It is closer to the middle of the body in aquatic snakes than in terrestrial or arboreal snakes, which have hearts typically 15% to 20% of the body length from the head. In wide-bodied animals, the heart may lay on either the right or left side of the coelomic cavity. In small snakes and nonconstrictors, the heart is the first round palpable structure caudal to the head. However, it is more difficult to palpate the heart in large constrictors, especially if the snake is obese. Anesthesia with an inhalant anesthetic may be necessary to provide adequate relaxation for cardiac venipuncture and is recommended in active animals to prevent injury. The reader should refer to the Danielle Strahl-Heldreth and Sathya K. Chinnadurai's article, "Ambulatory Anesthesia for the Exotic Veterinary Practitioner," in this issue for further details. The heart can be identified with either a Doppler flow detection apparatus or ultrasound machine if palpation is inadequate. Once located, the heart is gently stabilized by placing a thumb below the apex of the ventricle and applying a slight cranial pressure. Use of other fingers to "hold" the heart may benefit stabilization. The needle is introduced cranially into the ventricle, at 45°, while a slight negative pressure is applied until blood flow is attained. The flow is pulsatile and the negative pressure should be released intermittently to allow cardiac chamber filling. Aspiration of clear fluid represents pericardial fluid. This sample may be collected for fluid analysis but is a contaminant in a blood sample that must be discarded. In such instances, the needle should be withdrawn, a new syringe and needle secured, and the procedure repeated. In obtaining samples from this location, the clinician may notice that blood can be withdrawn with each heartbeat. After a maximum of 3 failed attempts at obtaining a blood sample from the heart, further sampling attempts should be discontinued.[9] When performed appropriately, this procedure has no morbidity or mortality.

The supravertebral (subcarapacial) vein is located in the midline below the anterior aspect of the carapace in chelonians. The needle is inserted where the skin joins the shell and advanced caudally until blood is aspirated. The vessel is usually located just above the posterior cervical vertebrae. This technique may require a long needle. This vessel closely approximates the spinal canal. If clear liquid is observed, in addition to the possibility of lymph, it may be cerebrospinal fluid.

The brachial vein is a plexus of vessels at the flexor surface of the elbow that may be accessible in lizards and chelonia. This site is particularly useful in large chelonians, especially tortoises. The animal is gently placed in dorsal recumbency and the leg extended forward either by the veterinary surgeon or by an assistant. The junction of the biceps tendon and the radius forms a V into which the needle is inserted. The needle is directed at an acute angle into the notch in small tortoises or at a perpendicular angle in large tortoises. Tilting the tortoise so that the leg used for venipuncture is dependent may help.

FIELD SAMPLE PROCESSING AND SUBMISSION

In general, the sample should be processed to stability immediately in the field. Blood smears should be made immediately and possibly PCV should be spun on site if a complete blood count is planned. Blood samples intended for biochemical analysis should be centrifuged immediately in the field. Power sources including outlets in boats or motorized vehicles as well as converters attached to batteries may be used for this purpose. If refrigeration or freezing is required to preserve a sample and this is not available, there is no reason to take the sample.

Anticoagulant choice is based on desired testing. Blood should be collected into microtainer tubes containing lithium heparin for biochemical analysis because serum, which lacks anticoagulant, may form a gel in a percentage of samples, especially those from animals with inflammatory disease, that is, the samples that you care about. For hematologic sampling, lithium heparin or in some species, dipotassium ethylenediaminetetraacetic acid (EDTA) may be used as an anticoagulant.[10] The use of EDTA can cause hemolysis in some species, especially chelonians.[11] The use of EDTA is suitable as an anticoagulant for snake blood.[12] In some reptiles, such as the green iguana, total white blood cell and differential counts are more similar to those of nonanticoagulated blood films in samples collected in EDTA versus those collected in heparin.[13] When heparin is used as an anticoagulant, a slight bluish or pink tinge in the background of blood films may be observed,[5] and leukocytes may not stain as intensely as those collected in EDTA (**Fig. 3**). These potential heparin effects can make the assessment of abnormal morphology such as toxic change difficult to impossible. Furthermore, leukocytes and thrombocytes often tend to clump more in heparinized blood than in EDTA-anticoagulated blood.[14] Cell clumping may adversely affect cell counts and the accuracy of the blood film evaluation. To avoid these artifacts, blood with no anticoagulant may be used to perform a blood film immediately after collection. Other anticoagulants that have been used for collection of whole blood include sodium heparin and ammonium heparin, which are used to heparinize the needle and syringe to prevent clot formation. There are new cell stabilizers, originally designed to stabilize delicate neoplastic cells, that have been explored in field samples from mammalian species that will likely aid in the stabilization of reptiles in the field. In a study by Molter and colleagues,[15] refrigerated koala blood was stabilized for 2 weeks, which has the benefit of enabling a complete blood count analysis for blood samples taken in remote areas. Further study in reptiles is warranted.

Anticoagulated samples for hematology that are found to have macroclots that can be found upon visual inspection will produce variably erroneous results. It is required in American Society for Veterinary Clinical Pathology guidelines that the clinician be

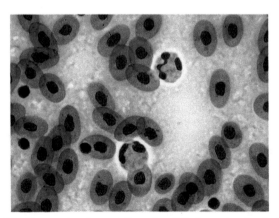

Fig. 3. Heparin artifact in a water dragon. Heparin artifact may be due to increased heparin concentration, increased protein concentration, or both. This water dragon's total solids were 7.8, so protein concentration was not significantly increased indicating that overheparinization in a small sample was likely a cause. Heparin binds the eosin Y stain in the Romanowsky stains to create the pink, sometimes granular, hue in the background. (*Modified* Wrights stain at 500× magnification).

contacted by the laboratory either in writing or by phone and informed that the sample will produce erroneous results. Because the varying degree of inaccuracy cannot be predicted, clotted samples are unsuitable for analysis and it is not recommended that these samples be analyzed.[2]

Blood samples submitted for a complete blood count should be accompanied by blood smears made immediately after collection. The blood smear can be stored for 5 to 7 days in a dark, cool place with no degradation. Longer storage of untreated blood smears is possible, but there may be degradation of staining properties. In the field, blood smears may be dipped in methanol (the light blue, first stain of Romanowsky stains including DiffQuik) for 30 seconds to 5 minutes for fixation and indefinite preservation. This step is important to a quality result in regions with either high humidity and heat or extreme cold. In addition to cell estimates, red blood cell and white blood cell morphology, including the presence of toxic changes, blood parasites, bacteria, and viral inclusions, can be assessed with the blood smear. Blood films made in the field or clinic should not be refrigerated and should be protected from condensation and freezing during transport to the laboratory.

PLASMA

Blood biochemical evaluation is performed using either plasma (anticoagulated blood that contains clotting factors) or serum (no anticoagulant with a lower protein concentration than plasma). Plasma is preferred because approximately one-third of serum samples form a proteinaceous gel that prevents analysis. Additionally, plasma may be separated immediately, thus preventing variable duration of cell exposure. Plasma will also have slightly more volume than serum samples, which may be important in obtaining results from smaller animals. It should be noted that injectable heparin is generally sodium heparin, which will falsely increase the concentration of sodium in the sample if added in any significant volume. Therefore, all visible droplets of injectable heparin should be thoroughly expelled before venipuncture. The blood sample should be centrifuged immediately and the plasma removed from the blood cells. Separation of plasma from small blood volumes is facilitated by the use of tubes containing plasma separators.

TISSUE COLLECTION

Bone marrow is not commonly collected from reptiles because most cytopenias are temperature induced. Aspiration is not possible due to the fibrous nature of reptilian tissues and lysis of the cells. Biopsy may be performed using a Jamshidi needle, which is generally used for bone biopsy. A 16-G needle is suitable in most moderately sized reptiles. Although bone marrow can be collected from bones of the appendicular skeleton of lizards, it is difficult to obtain in snakes. Further, in adult to geriatric reptiles there may be very little active bone marrow. Bone marrow in adult chelonians may only be present in some portions of the flat bones of the carapace and is perhaps most easily collected in the gular region.

Biopsy samples are collected for histopathology, polymerase chain reaction (PCR), or other molecular diagnostic testing, culture, and electron microscopy. Histologic interpretation depends on the preservation of normal cell and tissue architecture, and the biopsy sample should be of sufficient size to allow interpretation. When possible, multiple samples should be collected, especially in large lesions where the center may be necrotic. Obvious overlying necrotic tissue may need to be removed to allow the collection of a diagnostic sample. The transition area between a lesion and apparently healthy tissue should always be sampled.

The most commonly used fixative is 10% buffered formalin. Other solutions may be required depending on the type of lesion and suspected cause, such as Bouin's fixative required for preservation of eyes. To investigate possible gout, a representative tissue sample should be placed in alcohol fixative, because uric acid crystals will dissolve in buffered formalin. Samples for electron microscopy are most commonly placed in 2% glutaraldehyde solution in a dark refrigerator. However, the desired preservation solution may vary with technique and electron microscopy technologist, so be sure to contact the laboratory before sample collection for electron microscopy.

Samples for PCR and culture should be collected aseptically and placed in sterile sealed containers. The samples should be refrigerated or frozen if there is likely to be a delay in processing. Biopsy samples are usually excellent for microbiological culture. The sample should always be collected aseptically and should be frozen for further evaluation when a virus or unusual infectious agent is suspected. Storage in formalin is not recommended for tissue specifically intended for molecular analysis or culture. PCR may be performed on tissue from paraffin blocks that have been stored for several years, provided that they did not spend more than 72 hours in formalin before paraffin embedding. There may be significant loss in sensitivity and false-negative results are common when tissues are not handled correctly for PCR.

Cytology is indicated to evaluate the number and types of cells present, as well as the presence of infectious agents. Special stains are indicated when fungi, protozoans, and typical and atypical (eg, Chlamydia) bacteria are suspected. It is important to preserve the integrity of any cells present in the samples, which can be difficult in the fibrotic lesions that typically lack a fluid component produced by reptiles. The caseated nature of inflammatory lesions and the fibrous nature of many masses preclude sampling by aspiration, especially with smaller than 20-G needles. Impression smears and scrapes generally yield more cells. A clean small paintbrush or a scalpel blade can be used for transferring samples directly from small lesions to a slide.

Impression smears are made by either touching a tissue sample to a glass slide or touching the slide to the lesion. To improve the quality of the sample, the surface is gently cleaned of blood, typically by dabbing the cut surface on an absorbent paper. The tissue is then gently touched to the slide in multiple places in a regular pattern. The smear can be stained and examined immediately, allowing an immediate diagnosis. The tissue or lesion may then be placed in formalin for routine histologic evaluation.

A scrape of a mass, organ, or lesion should be performed in the active, parenchymal area. Necrotic regions as well as organ or mass capsules generally yield nondiagnostic samples and should be avoided. The region of interest can be scraped with the blunt or sharp edge of a scalpel blade and gently spread onto a glass slide. If the smear is thick, a second slide should gently be placed on top and a pull preparation created. The smear is air dried and then stained.

A fine needle aspirate is obtained by inserting a needle into the tissue or lesion. Ultrasound guidance facilitates accurate needle placement in the abnormal target tissue. Sample collection may be accomplished using a vacuum created by an attached syringe or more gently by redirecting the needle several times through the lesion (ie, the stab technique). A stab technique works well for most masses, especially vascular masses. The authors usually use an 18- or 20-G hypodermic needle attached to a 3- to 12-mL syringe. Negative pressure is repetitively generated in the syringe, by pulling on the plunger, while the needle is redirected within the lesion. If an excessive amount of blood is collected, the needle is withdrawn and a new needle and syringe used. Even if no tissue seems to have been collected in the syringe, the needle is disconnected, the plunger drawn back, and reconnected, and any trapped material in the needle blown on to the slide. The aspirate is then gently expressed on to a slide and a pull preparation is made using a second slide or coverslip. Aspirates can also be obtained through the side port of an endoscope using a flexible cannula.

Unfixed cytologic specimens and air-dried, unstained cytology smears should be protected from exposure to formalin and formalin fumes, which interfere with subsequent staining, by shipping in tightly sealed containers or shipping separately from formalin-fixed biopsy specimens. Similar to blood smears, cytology smears should be protected from humidity and temperature extremes. Identification of the site, method, and time of collection is of great importance in optimal interpretation and diagnostic result.

URINE AND FLUID COLLECTION

Chelonians and some lizards (eg, green iguana) possess bladders. In these animals, the ureters do not empty directly into the bladder but close to the area where the bladder neck connects to the cloaca. Urine samples may be collected by cystocentesis, potentially using ultrasound guidance to identify the bladder. Samples collected by cystocentesis should not be treated as aseptic. Interpretation of reptile urinalysis is made difficult by the mixing of renal and gastrointestinal (and occasionally reproductive) excretions in the cloacal region.[8]

Urine is a caustic sample in all species and urinalysis should be performed within 1 hour, although the American Society for Veterinary Clinical Pathology guidelines allow up to a 24-hour window for some constituents. Identification of the urine collection method is important when interpreting the presence and concentration of potential contaminants, including blood and bacteria. The collector should clearly state the method by which the urine was obtained, such as catheterization, cystocentesis, or from the floor or cage.[16]

If immediate examination is not possible, urine should be stored at refrigerated temperatures to minimize changes in urine physical and chemical composition and to inhibit bacterial growth. Urine should be protected from exposure to ultraviolet light to prevent degradation. Lids should be secure to prevent evaporation and/or volatilization of urine constituents (eg, ketones). Strict recommendations for the duration of refrigerated storage cannot be made, because this factor depends on specific urine components.[17] Storage for a maximum of 24 hours in the refrigerator is generally recommended (Osborne cautiously suggests 6–8 hours), but urine may be stable for shorter or longer periods depending on its initial makeup. Chemical constituents that are particularly unstable include bilirubin and glucose, and pH if bacteria are present.[17,18] Stability of formed elements depends on urine pH and concentration. Crystals may form in vitro during storage at either room temperature or under refrigeration.[18,19] If crystalluria is a clinical concern, freshly collected urine should be examined immediately. Refrigerated samples should be brought to room temperature before analysis. Because urinalysis results may be affected by storage duration and temperature, the time the urine was collected, the time it arrived in the laboratory, and method of storage should be recorded. Alternative methods of preservation are available for stabilization of urine chemistry, inhibition of bacterial growth, and preservation of formed elements in mammalian urine. Referral laboratories and manufacturers should be contacted for up-to-date recommendations. Manufacturer's claims should be followed regarding intended use of particular preservative and duration of storage.

Normal urine has a clear to light yellow fluid component, with a white to light yellow urate component. Its specific gravity is generally lower than in mammalian species, and both the bladder and cloaca modify urine, so it is not necessarily reflective of what is happening in the kidneys. Normal urine sediment is composed of uric acid precipitates, sloughed squamous epithelial cells, less than 5 white and less than 5 red blood cells per 40× field, and low quantities of (predominantly Gram-negative) bacteria. Motile and nonmotile protozoans are occasionally observed in low numbers in normal reptilian urine. Many of these are believed to be intestinal commensals; however, some protozoans, such as amebae and *Hexamita*, are true pathogens.

For fluid samples, 1 or more direct smears should be made from the fluid sample before any concentration or fixation procedures are performed. The smears can be stained or left unstained and should be submitted with the fluid sample. This step will allow for an estimation of the cell count and proportions of various cell types. This may provide valuable information that influences the cytologic interpretation and provides additional quality control by enabling the cytopathologist to ensure that the cell counts match estimates made from these smears. This process also avoids the situation in which extreme cell density of concentrated samples prevents optimal cytologic evaluation. Sedimented, air-dried samples are also recommended especially in from fluids, which seem to be clear.

Cavity washes are used to collect samples from the upper and lower gastrointestinal and respiratory tracts, and the coelomic cavity. Samples collected from a wash may be evaluated for cells and the presence of infectious agents, including bacteria (via aerobic and anaerobic bacterial culture and Gram staining), fungi (via culture and special stains), parasites, and viral inclusions. Use sterile isotonic solutions to preserve cytologic integrity and prevent tissue injury. Before drying and staining, a portion of the sample should always be examined as a wet mount to look for the presence of motile protozoan and other parasites.

A tracheal wash is performed when respiratory disease is suspected (**Fig. 4**). To obtain an uncontaminated sample, the trachea is intubated with a sterile endotracheal tube and a sterile catheter passed through it into the respiratory tract. Chemical immobilization is necessary for endotracheal tube placement. Approximately 1 to 5 mL/kg of isotonic fluid

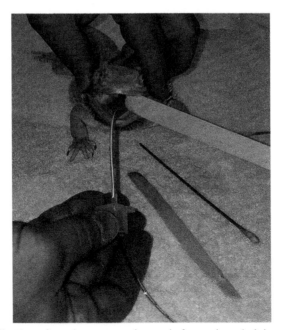

Fig. 4. Sterile collection of a pulmonary wash sample from a bearded dragon (*Pogona vitticeps*) under anesthesia. (*Courtesy of* Adolf Maas, DVM, Bothell, WA.)

is then introduced and rapidly aspirated. This step may have to be repeated several times to obtain a diagnostic sample. Positioning the animal to allow gravity to assist fluid flow will facilitate a good sample collection. Endoscopy may be used to assist in collecting and mucopurulent or lesional material. The most useful diagnostic material is often contained in the distal portion of the catheter and should not be discarded. Endoscopy may also be used to assist in bronchoalveolar lavage from larger animals.[20]

Gastrointestinal washes are performed similarly to a tracheal wash in the anesthetized animal, but the volume of fluid is increased. Gastric washes may be difficult in snakes because the stomach extends over one-half of the length of the body from the head.

Cloacal washes are usually performed when a reptile has not defecated recently and a fecal sample is required for cytologic and parasitic examination. A large flexible urinary catheter is inserted into the cloaca and/or colon and an isotonic electrolyte solution infused and aspirated. In snakes and some other lizards there is a large ventral scale that protects the cloaca like a flap. This flap needs to be gently elevated before a catheter can be directed cranially into the cloaca. The collected material is centrifuged at 3000 rpm for 5 minutes, the liquid decanted and the sediment used for analysis. A portion of the sediment is immediately placed under a coverslip and examined for evidence of motile protozoans and parasite ova. A pull preparation should be made from the sediment samples, air dried, and stained for cytologic and bacterial examination.

Reptiles do not have the subarachnoid space from which mammalian cerebrospinal fluid (CSF) samples are collected. Many reptiles are too small for any sample to be collected. In species greater than 0.75 kg, 0.2 mL of CSF may be collected from the subdural space, which is found between the pia–arachnoid layer that lines the surface of the brain and spinal cord, and the dura mater. Because the spinal cord extends to the very end of the tail tip in reptiles, CSF samples are best collected at the junction between the occiput and the first cervical vertebra. The site is cleaned with appropriately diluted chlorhexidine. A hypodermic needle (attached to a 2-mL syringe) is inserted midline at a 90° angle to the skin surface, and advanced slowly. A slight pop is felt when entering the subdural space and CSF starts to flow freely. The 3 layers encountered in the occipital sinus are lymph, blood, and CSF. Care should be taken to avoid excessive retraction of the syringe plunger because this motion will result in damage to the underlying nervous tissue. Samples should be examined microscopically immediately, because cellular deterioration occurs quickly in heparin. Avoid placement of CSF in EDTA tubes used in mammalian CSF analysis because lysis of the sample may result in short periods of time.[8]

TOXICOLOGY

The diagnosis of heavy metal toxicosis requires whole blood collected in mineral-free tubes and tissue, usually liver, evaluation. It is recommended that a veterinary toxicologist be contacted to determine appropriate sample submission based on possible causes. Reptiles seem to be very resistant to some toxins and the significance of a tissue or blood level cannot necessarily be related to clinical effects in a mammal.

Lead poisoning may be caused by the ingestion of fishing sinkers, pieces of metal, hunting pellets, and other objects.[21] Clinical symptoms are less well-documented than in mammals, and crocodilians seem to be able to deal with lead levels that would be rapidly fatal in a mammal. High blood lead levels have been reported in a common snapping turtle (3.6 ppm; normal, <0.6 ppm),[22] and a spur-thighed tortoise (1.89 μmol/L; avian normal, <1.2 μmol/L[21]), although the correlation with clinical signs was limited. Treatment consists of removal of lead from the digestive tract and chelation with sodium calcium edetate (10–40 mg/kg intramuscularly every 24 hours, tapering the dose as blood lead levels decrease).

BACTERIA

Material for culture should be collected before beginning antimicrobial therapy. All specimens should be transported in labeled, tightly sealed, leak-proof containers that are not externally contaminated. Aspirates of lesions are preferable to swabs due to a lesser degree of contamination. If swabs are to be used, minitip culturettes may enable the practitioner to swab the area of interest more precisely or pierce a lesion to take a deeper sample. Swabs may also be moistened with sterile fluid so that bacteria and cells do not adhere to the fibers.

The selection of the appropriate transport media is essential for useful culture results. Less fastidious organisms, such as pseudomonad and coliform bacteria, are relatively hardy and can be expected to survive overnight transport at room temperature on a standard collection swab such as Stuart's or Amies transport medium. For noncoliform bacteria, Amies is preferable. Anaerobic samples should be placed immediately into anaerobic transport media, such as thioglycollate agar. More fastidious organisms require specific transport media. Samples for *Mycoplasma* should immediately be placed into a mycoplasma culture broth such as SP4 or Frey's. Because mycoplasmas lack cell walls, they are highly susceptible to desiccation. If the sample is taken with a swab, the chances for successful culture are greatly improved by premoistening swabs in sterile mycoplasma broth or other sterile isotonic solution. Many mycoplasmas are slow growing, and it may take several weeks to obtain culture results. It is recommended to discuss your suspicion with your laboratory. Concurrent serology and PCR are recommended if mycoplasmal disease is suspected, as clinically warranted. Serum samples for serology should be shipped refrigerated or frozen in tightly sealed, leak-proof containers that are not externally contaminated. It should be noted that single sample, positive serology on provides information on disease exposure, not causation of clinical signs. *Chlamydia* cultures also require specialized transport media, which should be provided by your laboratory if they can culture this organism. If the sample is taken with a premoistened swab, the chances for a successful culture are greatly improved. Concurrent PCR may be needed in the face of negative culture if disease associated with *Chlamydia* is suspected.[8] Although caution should be used in any laboratory that defines their assays as research based and not diagnostic, this author recommends identification with concurrent sequencing at the Zoo Med Diagnostic Laboratory at the University of Florida. A submission form link may be found here http://labs.vetmed.ufl.edu/available-tests/zoo-med-infections/.

Mycobacterial or actinomycete cultures are often most successful from biopsy samples. Tissue samples may be sent directly to the laboratory in a sterile sealed container. Mycobacteria are very slow growing and culture results may take up to several months. This author recommends National Jewish Health Mycobacteriology Laboratory for culture of this difficult organism. A sample submission form may be found here at the laboratory's website https://www.nationaljewish.org/treatment-programs/directory/mycobacteriology. Concurrent histology with acid-fast staining is recommended if mycobacterial or nocardial disease is suspected.

Blood culture is indicated when bacteria is identified on blood smear and is not a stain contaminant. Bacteremia is more common in reptiles than in mammals or birds, and blood culture can be useful for identifying an organism causing lesions in solid tissues. The skin at the venipuncture site must be aseptically prepared, which may take numerous cleansings especially if the tail veins is used. The needle should be changed and the bottle wiped with alcohol before placing the sample in the blood culture bottle. Pediatric blood culture bottles are available and require smaller samples. Although it is ideal to sample the volume recommended by the manufacturer of the culture bottle, collecting such a volume may be contraindicated by the size of smaller patients. A culturette may be saturated with blood in low-volume samples with successful culture of the pathogen.

Many infectious microorganisms that afflict reptiles grow best at lower temperatures than do mammalian infectious agents and require longer culture times. Many standard veterinary microbiology facilities established for the culture of mammalian organisms do not have knowledgebase or may not be equipped to deal with these differences. The reptilian practitioner must therefore be knowledgeable about and have a good relationship with the microbiology laboratory management to ensure correct culture of organisms. For example, samples may need to be cultured at a variety of temperatures to elicit growth, depending on the life patter of the reptile. Additionally, many if not all bacterial identification kits for laboratories are developed around organisms likely to be found in mammals or birds. If an identification seems to be unusual, it is appropriate to discuss the result with a microbiologist.

Both aerobic and anaerobic bacteria are common causes of disease in reptiles. They are also a normal part of the fauna of the gastrointestinal and upper respiratory tracts, as well as the skin. Consequently, culture alone may be insufficient to make a causal association, and results need to be correlated with histopathology or cytology. Samples commonly submitted for bacterial culture include swabs from body orifices or lesions, cavity washes, tissue aspirates, blood cultures, and biopsy samples. Many bacteria have not been successfully cultured, and for organisms such as *Chlamydia* spp., *Mycoplasma* spp, or *Mycobacterium* spp., consensus PCR- and sequencing-based diagnostics should be considered if the organisms are suspected in the face of negative culture.

SUMMARY

Diagnostic test results are only as good as the quality of the sampling, storage, transport, and laboratory analysis. The practitioner must not only make the correct selection of diagnostic tests to analyze, but in the veterinary clinic, must also be vigilant to insure that degraded samples do not produce invalid results. Although these tasks may be challenging, it is ultimately rewarding because quality diagnostic results equal accurate diagnoses, thus, providing the best possible treatment leading to the health of the patient.

REFERENCES

1. Flatland B, Freeman KP, Friedrchs KR, et al. ASVCP quality assurance guidelines: control of general analytical factors in veterinary laboratories. Vet Clin Pathol 2010;39:264–77.
2. Vap LM, Harr KE, Arnold JE, et al. ASVCP quality assurance guidelines: control of preanalytical and analytical factors in veterinary laboratories related to hematology for mammalian and non-mammalian species, hemostasis, and crossmatching. Vet Clin Pathol 2011;41:8–17.
3. Anderson NL, Wack RF, Hatcher R. Hematology and clinical chemistry reference ranges for clinically normal, captive New Guinea snapping turtle (Elseya novaeguineae) and the effects of temperature, sex and sample type. J Zoo Wildl Med 1997;28:394–403.
4. MacLean GS, Lee AK, Withers PC. Hematological adjustments with diurnal changes in body temperature in a lizard and a mouse. Comp Biochem Physiol A Comp Physiol 1975;51:241–9.

5. Stacy NI, Harr KE. Reptile clinical pathology. In: Jacobson ER, editor. Infectious diseases and pathology of reptiles. 2nd edition. Boca Raton (FL): CRC Press; 2018. p. 167–83.
6. Wright RK, Cooper EL. Temperature effects on ectotherm immune responses. Dev Comp Immunol 1981;(5 Suppl):117–22.
7. Ottaviani G, Tazzi A. The lymphatic system. In: Gans C, Parsons TS, editors. Biology of the reptilia, vol. 6. New York: Academic Press; 1977. p. 315–462.
8. Heard DH. Diagnostic sampling and laboratory tests. In: Girling SJ, Raiti R, editors. BSAVA manual of reptiles. London: BSAVA; 2004. p. 71–86.
9. Jacobson E. Blood collection techniques in reptiles: laboratory investigations. In: Fowler ME, editor. Zoo and wild animal medicine. Current therapy 3. Philadelphia: WB Saunders Co; 1993. p. 144–52.
10. Harr KE, Raskin RE, Heard DJ. Temporal hematologic and biochemical effects of three commonly used anticoagulants on macaw (Ara sp.) and Burmese python (python molurus bivittatus) blood. Vet Clin Pathol 2005;34:383–8.
11. Muro J, Cuenca R, Pastor J, et al. Effects of lithium heparin and tripotassium EDTA on hematologic values of Hermann's tortoises (Testudo hermanni). J Zoo Wildl Med 1998;29:40–4.
12. Salakij C, Salakij J, Apibal S, et al. Hematology, morphology, cytochemical staining, and ultrastructural characteristics of blood cells in king cobras (Ophiophagus hannah). Vet Clin Pathol 2002;31:116–26.
13. Hanley CS, Hernandez-Divers SJ, Bush S, et al. Comparison of the effect of dipotassium ethylenediaminetetraacetic acid and lithium heparin on hematologic values in the green iguana (Iguana iguana). J Zoo Wildl Med 2004;35:328–32.
14. Hawkey CM, Dennett TB. A colour atlas of comparative veterinary haematology. London: Wolfe Publishing Ltd; 1989.
15. Molter CM, Harr KE, Zaback M, et al. Streck cell preservative stabilizes koala (Phascolarctos cinereus) whole blood for complete blood counts. J Zoo Wildl Med 2018.
16. Gunn-Christie RG, Flatland B, Friedrichs KR, et al. Preanalytical, analytical, and postanalytical factors for clinical chemistry, urinalysis, and cytology in veterinary laboratories. Vet Clin Pathol 2011;41:18–26.
17. Rabinovitch A, Arzoumanian L, Curcio KM, et al. Urinalysis; approved guideline. 3rd edition. Wayen (MI, IL): Clinical Laboratory Standards Institute; 2009. Document.
18. Albasan H, Lulich JP, Osborne CA, et al. Effects of storage time and temperature on pH, specific gravity, and crystal formation in urine samples from dogs and cats. J Am Vet Med Assoc 2003;222:176–9.
19. Sturgess. 2001.
20. LaFortune M, Gobel T, Jacobson E, et al. Respiratory bronchoscopy of subadult American alligators (Alligator mississippiensis) and tracheal wash evaluation. J Zoo Wildl Med 2005;36:12–20.
21. Chitty JR. Lead toxicosis in a Greek tortoise (Testudo graeca). Proceedings of the Association of Reptilian and Amphibian Veterinarians, 101. Minneapolis (MN), 2003.
22. Borkowski R. Lead poisoning and intestinal perforations in a snapping turtle (Chelydra serpentina) due to fishing gear ingestion. J Zoo Wildl Med 1997;28: 109–13.

Ambulatory Anesthesia for the Exotic Veterinary Practitioner

Danielle Strahl-Heldreth, MS, DVM[a],
Sathya K. Chinnadurai, DVM, MS, DACZM, DACVAA[b],*

KEYWORDS

- Ambulatory • Anesthesia • Avian • Exotic • Reptile • Small mammal

KEY POINTS

- Anatomic nuances that make intubation, intravenous access, and monitoring challenging are critical factors to understand before attempting to anesthetize a new species, especially in remote locations.
- Adaptation of anesthetic monitoring devices designed for humans and domestic animals to exotic animals is challenging but necessary for safe field anesthesia.
- Literature regarding anesthesia in companion exotic animal species continues to grow, emphasizing the importance of safe anesthesia and reliable anesthetic monitoring.
- Routinely used inhalant delivery devices can be modified for field/portable use for exotic animal patients; commercially manufactured portable machines are also available.
- Remote capture equipment is often needed for field anesthesia of large or dangerous exotic animals, so practitioners are cautioned to train and seek experienced instruction before attempting to use these devices on patients.

INTRODUCTION

With the growing popularity in the ownership of nontraditional species, there is a growing need for veterinarians to be able to provide out-of-clinic health assessments on privately owned exotic species. Ambulatory (field/portable) anesthesia is often required for diagnostic and surgical procedures in remote or nonhospital settings. Anesthesia for diagnostic procedures is commonly used to ensure the safety of personnel and exotic veterinary patients, particularly in instances when there is an inability to transport the animal to the clinic owing to logistical or safety reasons. Often, the stress associated with handling even for the most minimally invasive procedures (ie, transport, physical examination, and blood collection) can result in injury from

Disclosure: The authors have nothing to disclose.
[a] University of Illinois College of Veterinary Medicine, Veterinary Teaching Hospital, 1008 W Hazelwood Drive, Urbana, IL 61821, USA; [b] Brookfield Zoo, Chicago Zoological Society, 3300 Golf Road, Brookfield, IL 60513, USA
* Corresponding author.
E-mail address: sathya.chinnadurai@czs.org

self-inflicted trauma or iatrogenically owing to struggling during restraint and handing. Performing heavy sedation or general anesthesia in the field is not without its difficulties and can be a source of stress for many veterinarians and their animal patients; even under the most ideal of circumstances, there is an increased risk of morbidity and mortality. This article focuses on the preparation of such an anesthetic event, as well as the implementation of ambulatory anesthesia in a host of privately owned exotic and wild animals.

PLANNING

Preparation in the perianesthetic period is paramount to ensure a safe and effective anesthetic event for both veterinary subjects and human clinicians. Whether it be for capture, surgery, examination, or treatment, the anesthetist should ascertain if the anesthesia is necessary and whether the benefits outweigh the potential risks to the animals and human personnel. If anesthesia is truly necessary, several factors must be considered during the perianesthetic period. When planning the anesthetic protocol, the ambulatory veterinarian should consider the species of interest, purpose of immobilization, and the procedural requirements including type and degree of restraint needed to provide safe capture and immobilization, as well as the environmental elements associated with the field setting (ie, temperature, terrain, bodies of water for terrestrial animals, and other hazards).

Species of Interest

It is important that the anesthetist has knowledge of the historical response of the species to restraint, capture, and immobilization. Drug protocol selection, doses and animal's response change between species and vary within species.[1] Therefore, the anesthetist must tailor the ambulatory anesthetic protocol to the species of interest, considering age, sex, body weight range, basic feeding habits, seasonal reproductive and condition cycles, habitat, and response to currently available drugs.

Herd animals such as wild equids, ungulates, and large birds (ostriches, emus) have an instinctual flight response to stressful situations, such as chase, capture, and confinement, which makes them more prone to self-trauma, collision, catastrophic fractures, and myopathies. Visual barriers or appropriately sized holding areas may help to decrease the flight distance and allow for closer access to animals. In contrast, large carnivores may choose to stand their ground in an aggressive manner if confronted with the likelihood of capture and restraint. For an assessment of a flock, aviary, or aquarium enclosure, it is important to consider the depth and height of the enclosure to allow for appropriate catch and release of individual animals.

The anesthetist must consider the likelihood of the animal's responses when developing a safe and effective anesthetic protocol. In many situations, remote drug delivery to an unrestrainable exotic animal is faster, less stressful, and with different, although no less deleterious, side effects, than physical restraint. Chase and capture techniques as well as extended periods of physical restraint have an increased risk of injury and mortality.

For the assessment of individual animals that are housed in a pair or group setting, it may be prudent to recommend an additional holding area be constructed to allow for the separation of animals when not immobilizing the group. For instance, many big cat hobbyists have multiple conspecific animals housed in the same enclosure. The ability to separate these animals is essential for both the safety of the animals and the human personnel. In herd animals, however, the premature separation of animals may be deleterious to the individuals that are housed separately for extended periods of time.

Patient Evaluation

Much like in a controlled, clinical setting, preanesthetic patient evaluation is a key step for a successful anesthetic event. In a free-ranging, large herd or multispecies setting, the anesthetist may not have the luxury of a complete medical history, physical examination, or preanesthetic diagnostics procedures. However, in a captive, semiwild, or zoologic setting, the anesthetist should rely on observational records regarding the overall health of the animal if a physical examination cannot be performed without the use of anesthesia.

The purpose of the patient evaluation depends partly on the reason for anesthesia. For diagnostic tests such as sampling from a diseased flock, herd or aquarium population, nontransportable carnivore, or when anesthesia is performed for management or conservation reasons, the patient evaluation may be done to eliminate individual animals that might be adversely affected by the procedure or to tailor the anesthetic protocol to the medical status of the individual animal.[2] In other cases, the injury or disease prompts intervention. A thorough preanesthetic evaluation allows the anesthetist to identify existing problems, predict complications, and design an anesthetic regimen to suit the needs of the individual patient and the procedure.

Additional Considerations

In addition to differences between species, there is also evidence to support differences in drug responses between sexes of the same species.[1,3] It is recommended that the anesthetist review both current and historical literature to help guide the drug protocol selection and adjust doses accordingly based on signalment of the individual animal being anesthetized.

The age and health status of the animal should also be taken into consideration when formulating an anesthetic plan. Young/juvenile, systemically healthy animals often require a higher dose of drug per unit body weight than adult animals.[4] Geriatric or debilitated animals often require less than animals within their prime life cycles.[5] Just as in domestic species in a clinic setting, there is a higher risk of anesthetic complications in older, debilitated animals. In addition, neonates often require a significant decrease in drug dosing.[4]

Environmental elements such as terrain and weather also play a significant role in planning and implementing a safe ambulatory anesthetic protocol, particularly when the animals are housed in an outdoor, unprotected area with minimal cover. In cases when an anesthetic event can be scheduled, it is recommended that the immobilization event take place in an optimal temperate, with freezing and sweltering temperatures avoided.[6]

Withdrawal of Food and Water

For many veterinary patients, an appropriate fasting time before giving anesthesia to prevent vomiting or regurgitation and subsequent aspiration of gastric contents is recommended.[7] However, neonates, birds, and small mammals are highly susceptible to hypoglycemic and are rarely fasted for more than 1 hour.[7] Stressed animals rarely eat or drink in the initial hours after capture and, thus, appropriate intraprocedural fluid therapy is recommended (see Supportive Care). The attending veterinarian should assess the biology of the animal involved and decide if a preanesthetic fasting and/or holding time is advisable and for what duration of time. Ideally, these decisions should be made during the planning phase of the event and can be relayed to the individuals charged with the animal's care.

DRUG DELIVERY ROUTES AND EQUIPMENT
Oral

The administration of drugs via an oral route can be a good alternative for premedicating stressed or fractious individual animals. However, drugs taken orally may have an altered rate of absorption, distribution, and clearance than when given by another route. These alterations in pharmacokinetics may result in prolonged induction and recovery times. The use of oral sedatives such as benzodiazepines, phenothiazines, and alpha-2 adrenergic agonists have been used in a wide range of species, including birds, miniature pigs, exotic carnivores, and nonhuman primates, for mild to moderate sedation.[8–13]

Intranasal

Intranasal administration of sedative and immobilization drugs has proven to be an easier and faster alternative than intravenous (IV) or intramuscular routes, respectively. It allows the administration of drugs to an awake animal that is retrained in a cage without the additional stress of physical restraint for injection. Protocols using alpha-2-adrenergic agonists and/or benzodiazepines have been reported in a wide range of veterinary patients, including cervids, pigs, and various bird species.[14–16] Owing to the close proximity necessary for the administration of these drugs, care must be taken to ensure that the possibility of accidental exposure is minimized with the use of face shield and/or other personal protective equipment.

Topical, Immersion, and Flow Techniques

With the growing number of fish and amphibian pets in private collections, it is important that veterinarians be skilled in the immobilization of these species. The implementation of immersion, topical, and flow anesthetic techniques is a good alternative for aquatic species including fish and amphibians.

Immersion is analogous to inhalant anesthesia in air breathing species and occurs when a diluted anesthetic is absorbed by the gills and/or skin to produce anesthesia. Fish are commonly anesthetized with immersion in respiratory anesthetic agents absorbed through the gills (eg, tricaine methanesulfonate, MS222, alphaxalone, and isoflurane), a technique that lacks the advantage of precision vaporizers used for these anesthetics used in air-breathing animals.[17] Advantages of immersion anesthesia include the lack of physical restraint necessary for induction, consistency in response, relatively high safety margin, and rapid recovery after removal to fresh water tank. The disadvantages of this technique include the relative difficulty in changing the anesthetic concentration in the water after the animal is immersed, the lack of stability for long procedures, and the irritating nature of some anesthetics that have been studied. Additionally, because fish and amphibian species are sensitive to environmental derangements, it is important to provide an oxygen supply while monitoring the pH, temperature, and mineral content of the anesthetic bath consistently throughout the anesthetic event.[18] It is recommended that water from the "home" tank be used for the anesthetic and recovery tanks whenever possible to help decrease the variability and potentially harmful effects of differences in these parameters.[18]

In cases where procedures are to be performed out of water or last more than a few minutes, it is recommended that recirculating or continuous flow anesthesia be implemented.[19] This method requires additional equipment and training. When using flow anesthesia, the induction of anesthesia is performed via the immersion method as discussed. When an appropriate level of anesthesia is reached, the animal can be transitioned to either a recirculating or nonrecirculating method for delivery of anesthesia.[19]

A classic recirculating delivery system uses a submersible pump that is placed within a container holding the anesthetic solution, and the anesthetic-filled water is pumped from this tank into the animal's mouth, over the gills, and out through the opercula.[19] The animal can be positioned on a moistened towel, sponge trough, or a fenestrated board above the anesthetic water tank so that the anesthetic media can be recirculated back to the anesthetic tank. This method is commonly used in larger fish and in field scenarios. The nonrecirculating method uses an IV fluid bag and fluid set as the anesthetic water reservoir and delivery method.[20] This method can be used for smaller fish species. For either of these methods, the flow rate is adjusted such that water flows into the mouth, gently over the gills, and out the opercula. Unsuitable flow rates can lead to inappropriate gas exchange or force water into the gastrointestinal tract.[20]

Hand-Held Injections

Hand-held injections for IV or intramuscular injections is the most direct method of drug administration. The successful completion of this technique requires cooperation of the animal or manual restraint. Care must be taken to ensure that the appropriately sized needle and syringe are used in such techniques to prevent harm to the animal (ie, tissue damage owing to trauma, needle breakage within animal) or drug loss.[1] While the hand injection route of drug administration comes with relatively few side effects to the animal, it is considered hazardous for the drug administrator. Trauma and wounds, include bites, kicks, and crushing injuries, inflicted by the restrained animal are common. Additional concerns of drug exposure through aerosolizing and self-injections are present; thus, the administration of ultrapotent opioids via hand injection to an awake animal is not recommended.[1]

Pole Syringes

Pole syringes are a means of drug administration to animals with the added safety of a long pole. This method allows the drug administrator to remain at a safe distance from the animal. Pole syringes were developed for use in animals that were confined within a small cage or chute but uncooperative or resistant to hand injection, or for instances when an animal was trapped in an area that did not allow for the administration of a hand injection.[1] This added distance for safety, however, comes with the price of control of the injection process, including the lack of control from animal movement and needle misdirection. This tool can be useful for administering an immobilizing dose of drugs or for "top-ups" to animals that are not completely immobilized, but approachable to within 0.5 to 2.0 m.[1]

There are a large variety of pole syringes currently in production by Dan-Inject, Safe-T-Flex, Tomahawk, and Zoolu. These devices range in syringe volume from 2.5 to 20.0 mL; however, it is generally recommended to limit the volume of drug for administration to less than 10 mL per administration site. The use of large-bore needles (16- to 18-G) on large (>30 kg) animals allows for the rapid administrations of large volumes of drug with less tissue damage from impact of remote delivery methods.[1] However, on smaller animals, it is recommended that the needle size be adjusted to 20- to 22-G needles to prevent serious injury. The muscle masses of the hindquarters are the preferred sites for drug administration when using this method of drug delivery. However, the shoulder muscle mass can be used in large animals.[1] Three types of pole syringes are currently available. The manual-pressure pole syringe is composed of a typical syringe body with an extended plunger to provide added length.[1] The force of depression of the plunger is based on the push against the resistance of the animal's body. A second type of pole syringe is engineered so that the extension pole is attached to the body of the syringe with a second, internal extension of the syringe plunger that is manually depressed to deposit the drug. The third type of pole syringe has a spring or gas pressure loaded plunger that is triggered when the needle presses on the animal's skin.[1]

REMOTE DRUG DELIVERY

Large exotic animal capture and immobilization often requires drug delivery to be performed over relatively long distances or "remotely." The use of remote delivery systems and darts, propelled by a variety of means, are the most practical methods of remotely delivery injectable drugs to animals that cannot be safely approached and handled. Darts can be projected via blowpipe, longbow, crossbows (which has fallen out of favor and is not discussed herein), compressed air projector, or gunpowder cartridge rifle.[1]

Darts

Darts, or projectile syringes, have 4 basic components, including a storage compartment, a method of injecting the drug (plunger), a needle to penetrate the skin, and a tailpiece or stabilizer for accurate flight. There are several dart types, which differ in the method in which the plunger is pushed forward to deliver the drug to the animal. The 3 most basic ways that this occurs is through either expansion of gas from an explosive charge, compressed air, or chemical reaction.[1]

Blowpipe or Blowgun

The blowpipe or blowgun are the recommended devices for the administration of small volumes of drugs at short to medium ranges (20–30 m).[1] There are 2 general types of blow pipes, the conventional lung-powered blow pipe and the compressed air or the CO_2-powered blow pipe. Both devices operate by the propelling a dart through a pipe either by rapid, controlled expulsion of the operator's breath or using compressed air or CO_2.[1] The effective range for the conventional blowpipe is limited (<20–30 m). Benefits include that blowpipes and guns are usually quiet and cause minimal trauma to the animal. These tools can be used on animals as small as 3 kg without concern. Powered blowpipes are preferred for delivering larger (3 mL) volumes over slightly longer distances (30 m).[1]

Dart Guns (Rifles and Pistols)

Dart guns (rifles and pistols) are the most widely used remote delivery system. These systems propel a dart using either the gas generated from compressed air, compressed CO_2, or a 0.22-caliber blank cartridge.[1] Dart guns are the most versatile of all the remote delivery systems with effective ranges up to 75 to 100 m depending on size of animal and target area.[1] Dart volumes can be larger; however, the larger the volume, the shorter the accurate range. Each of the 3 types of dart propulsion systems has advantages and disadvantages that should be studied before use in any immobilization event. Proper education of firearm safety and handling is recommended before the use of these systems.

TYPES OF ANESTHETIC PROTOCOLS

The ideal drug combination for an ambulatory anesthetic event should incorporate the properties of rapid onset of activity and a high margin of safety for the animal and human personnel. In a remote setting, it is also important to consider whether the drugs in combination can be antagonized and the stability of the drugs, particularly in different environmental conditions.

The pharmacology, benefits, and disadvantages of each possible drug protocol can be found in textbooks and publications, and are beyond the scope of this article.[1,6] Investigators should consult the available relevant literature related to the species of interest in their development of an immobilization protocol. In addition to the historical literature, the veterinarian should apply the criteria of drug availability, safety for the animal and human personnel, previous results in the species under investigation, the duration of effect required, the need for a reversal or antidote, and the legislative implications of using the drug (particularly in consumable species).

The 2 general categories of anesthetic agents are inhaled or injectable agents. Because field anesthesia needs to be simple, safe, effective, and transportable, injectable anesthesia is often used instead of inhalant anesthesia for logistical reasons, because the use of volatile inhalant anesthesia in the field is a tradeoff between the rapid induction and recovery associated with inhalants and the logistical difficulty of moving compressed gas cylinders and vaporizers into the field. However, solely injectable protocols lack the inherent ability of inhalants for fine tuning by means of incremental adjustments in depth. The injectable-only protocol also has an increased possibility of prolonged drug effect and renarcotization.

Inhalant Agents

Inhalant anesthetics are widely used in a clinical setting and possess unique advantages and disadvantages for use in an ambulatory setting (**Fig. 1**).[7] The most commonly used inhalants, isoflurane and sevoflurane, have been used in clinical and ambulatory settings. Inhalants anesthetics are administered and expelled via the respiratory system, which allows for a rapid and precise adjustment of the anesthetic depth of the patient. Disadvantages include the need to transport volatile fluids, expensive and cumbersome vaporizers, and logistical concerns of transporting compressed gases.[21] In addition, all current inhalant anesthetics are known to cause a

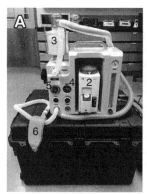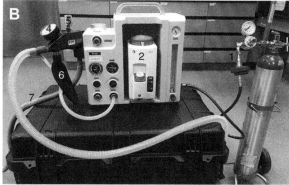

Fig. 1. Commercially available portable anesthesia machine. With labeled schematic of the components. This machine may be set up as a rebreather (A) and a nonrebreather (B). The components of the system include an (1) oxygen tank and regulator (visible in B only), (2) vaporizer, (3) carbon dioxide adsorbent canister (rebreathing system only), (4) pressure manometer, (5) adjustable pressure limiting (pop-off) valve, (6) rebreathing bag, and (7) scavenge hosing. (*From* Chinnadurai SK. Vaporizers and field anesthesia equipment for free-ranging wildlife. In: Miller E, Lamberski N, Calle P, editors. Fowler's zoo and wild animal medicine. 9th edition. St Louis (MO): Elsevier Saunders; 2018; p.177–184; with permission.)

dose-dependent decreases in cardiac output and blood pressure, which can be life threatening without appropriate monitoring and treatment. Additionally, the use of inhalants as a sole anesthetic agent is not recommended in several species, such as ungulate, bovid, and equids, because members of these species may exhibit turbulent, uncoordinated recoveries, which may lead to catastrophic injuries.[7] A review of the use of these agents in the species of interest is recommended before administration.

Injectable Anesthetics

Propofol is an ultrashort-acting injectable anesthetic that is labeled solely for IV administration. It is considered a sedative-hypnotic that lacks analgesic properties. Common, dose-dependent side effects of this drug include hypotension, apnea, and respiratory depression. Intubation and ventilatory support should be readily available if apnea occurs.[22] Alfaxalone, a neuroactive steroid, is an injectable anesthetic that can also be administered via the IV route. Like propofol, there are no analgesic properties. Unlike propofol, alfaxalone is considered to have a wide safety margin with little to no cardiovascular or respiratory depression seen with administration and can be administered via an intramuscular injection in several non-US countries.[22] Neither propofol nor alfaxalone are appropriate sole agents for painful procedures and additional analgesic drugs should be used.

Ketamine, a fast-acting dissociative anesthetic, is commonly used in clinical and ambulatory settings. This agent is often used in combination with a sedative, usually a benzodiazepine or alpha-2 agonist. Immobilizations with combinations including ketamine often have a characteristically rapid onset of action, immobilization within 10 minutes, and a long duration of action (up to 2 hours).[7] Ketamine provides excellent somatic analgesia, but poor visceral analgesia, and should not be used as the sole analgesic for procedures expected to cause visceral pain. When used alone or in higher doses, side effects include increased muscle tone, hyperthermia, excessive salivation, catecholamine release, and convulsions. Ketamine has no known antagonist; it is, therefore, recommended that it be used in combination with a reversible drug, particularly in field immobilization scenarios.[7]

Alpha-2 adrenergic agonists are commonly used in many immobilization combinations.[7] These potent central nervous system depressants, when administered alone, do not produce general anesthesia. However, this class of drugs is often used because it possesses sedative, muscle relaxant, and analgesic properties. When combined with opioids or dissociative anesthetics, such as ketamine, these drugs help to provide reliable anesthesia.[7] A dose-dependent depression of the respiratory (hypoxemia) and circulatory (hypertension and bradycardia) systems is also noted with these drugs when administered at higher dosages. Alpha-2 agonists can be reversed with the appropriate alpha-2 adrenergic antagonist to provide a smooth and fast recovery.[7]

Tiletamine-zolazepam is a commercial combination of a dissociative anesthetic and a benzodiazepine sedative and is widely used in veterinary medicine. This drug combination provides a smooth induction, good muscle relaxation, and analgesia when the appropriate dosages are administered. Tiletamine-zolazepam can be administered both IV and intramuscularly; however, caution is recommended with the IV route of administration. Considered a partially reversible combination, the zolazepam can be antagonized with flumazenil.[7]

Opioids have been used extensively in the immobilization of domestic and exotic species. These drugs are relatively fast acting, and provide both analgesia and sedation.[7] However, unlike alpha-2 agonists, they lack the muscle relaxation properties and are, therefore, commonly used in combination with other anesthetic agents. Common side effects seen with opioid combinations include excitation, muscle rigidity, regurgitation, severe respiratory depression and hypoxemia, and renarcotization. Most opioids used in a remote setting are ultrapotent and should be handled appropriately to decrease the chance of accidental human exposure. The appropriate opioid antagonist should be on hand for rapid reversal of the immobilization of the animal and for any accidental human exposure in the perianesthetic event.[7]

SPECIFIC ANESTHETIC PROTOCOLS AND DOSAGES

Owing to the limitations of this publication, the authors recommend that the reader refer to the textbooks: *Handbook of Wildlife Chemical Immobilization*, *Zoo and Wildlife Anesthesia and Immobilization* and *Veterinary Anesthesia and Analgesia* for specific anesthetic protocols based on species of interest.[1,23]

Once Immobilized

Once the animal can be safely approached and handled, there are several steps that should be taken to ensure a safe immobilization.

Body position and handling

Proper positioning of the anesthetized animal is essential for an uneventful anesthetic event. The anesthetist should note the position of the animal immediately after it becomes recumbent. Once the patient is deemed to be safe to approach and handle, its position should be manipulated when necessary.

It is important to ensure that the animal can breathe appropriately. Any obstacles or positions that impinge on respirations should be avoided, the neck should be positioned straight, and the nasal and oral cavities should be removed of debris. Most anesthetized animals should be positioned in sternal recumbency and the head should be elevated to a higher point than the body with the nose downward pointing to help prevent regurgitation and aspiration. Keep the animal on a flat surface to avoid pressure neuropathy or impairment of circulation.[1]

Once the animal is deemed to be in an appropriate position, a thorough physical examination should be performed. Keep eyes covered to reduce stimulation and protection from ultraviolet rays and debris. The ears may also be plugged with cotton to further prevent stimulation by loud sounds.[1] The eyes and ears should be thoroughly examined before implementation of these measures. Physical examination should include the central nervous, cardiovascular, and pulmonary systems, and, whenever possible, the heart rate, rhythm, pulse quality, and presence of a murmur; mucus membrane color and capillary refill time; hydration status; respiratory rate and rhythm; and overall demeanor and body condition should all be recorded.[1] If possible, an accurate body weight should also be obtained. In cases when preanesthetic weight cannot be measured, an animal should be weighed during anesthesia to allow for accurate dosing of supplemental or emergency drugs and retrospective calculation of the drug doses administered.

Monitoring

Reliable anesthetic monitoring is essential in both the clinical and field setting.[7] Although the most basic forms of anesthetic monitoring consist of measurements of heart rate, pulse quality, respiratory rate, and body temperature and can be carried out by the anesthetist with the use of their eyes, ears, a stethoscope, and a rectal thermometer, more advanced monitoring equipment is now available for field use. Ideally, monitoring of oxygenation, ventilation, and blood pressure should be performed on megavertebrate species during an immobilization event. Although pulse oximeters, capnography units, portable electrocardiograms, and Doppler or oscillometric blood pressure monitors are considered the standard of care monitoring in a clinical setting, certain modifications may be needed for ambulatory anesthetic monitoring[7] (**Fig. 2**).

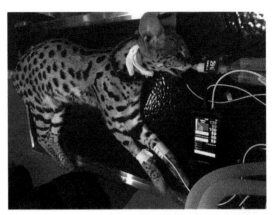

Fig. 2. Field anesthesia performed on an adult serval (*Leptailurus serval*). The animal was anesthetized with a combination of ketamine, midazolam, and dexmedetomidine and is being maintained on isoflurane, using a portable anesthesia machine. The animal is being monitored with battery powered pulse oximetry, noninvasive blood pressure, and capnography. In addition, the animal has both intravenous access and endotracheal intubation.

Before any anesthetic procedure, a plan for appropriate monitoring should be developed. This plan should be based on the anesthetic risk to the animal based on the species at hand, the anesthetic drugs selected, the proposed procedures, the environment and terrain, and the anticipated complications. The remote setting of ambulatory anesthesia often dictates the limitations of equipment and personnel that are available for patient monitoring during the anesthetic event. Ideally, monitoring of the cardiovascular and respiratory systems should be continuous with intermittent recordings of the parameters every 5 to 10 minutes on a designated anesthetic record. In addition to these continuously monitored parameters, the anesthetic depth and temperature should be monitored intermittently.[7]

In addition to the standard monitoring of physiologic parameters, several biochemical parameters should to be monitored in a field capture scenario. Blood glucose, systemic lactate, and or blood gases can be easily assessed with point-of-care portable analyzers. These measurements in conjunction with other monitoring techniques allow an overall assessment of the animal, including cardiopulmonary stability, tissue perfusion, and the likelihood of intraprocedural or postcapture complications.[7]

Supportive Care

Supportive care techniques for an ambulatory anesthetic event should be implemented based on the physiologic and biochemical monitoring values.

Intubation

Endotracheal intubation of air-breathing animals is desirable when undergoing surgical procedures. In addition to those undergoing surgery, it is recommended that animals that have an increased risk of regurgitation and respiratory compromise (such as hypoventilation) are intubated. However, depending on the anesthetic protocol used and the danger potential of the animal, it may not be necessary or possible to intubate safely.[7] Thus, the decision to intubate should be based on the well-being of the patient and the safety of the human personnel. If intubation is practical, the act of intubation should be performed by a veterinarian who has experience with the species and with the appropriate equipment, because trauma to the trachea and upper airway can result in serious consequences, ranging from hemorrhage and inflammation to subsequent tracheal stricture and death.[7] Even if intubation is not used routinely on every patient, having appropriately sized endotracheal tubes and a manual breathing unit (AMBU bag) available in every immobilization event is important to allow rapid correction of apnea or hypoventilation.[7]

Catheterization and fluid therapy

Intravascular access, when feasible, is recommended to facilitate supportive and emergency treatments during an anesthetic event. In some species, vascular access can prove challenging, something that may be compounded in a nonclinical setting. The difficulty in gaining vascular access is both time consuming and may outweigh the benefit of an expeditious completion of the procedure and recovery, the anesthetic team should assess whether IV catheters will be placed routinely or only during emergencies is another decision that should be made before the anesthetic event.[7]

The rational for fluid therapy should be based on the species, anesthetic protocol, reason for immobilization, and logistical constraints of the remote setting. For example, for patients that are anesthetized with anesthetic agents that cause hypotension, such as inhalants, a means of pressure support and fluid therapy is recommended to help maintain appropriate blood pressure. Similarly, if a surgical procedure is expected to result in significant blood loss or is very invasive, fluid therapy is essential.[7]

Analgesia

Just as in a clinical setting, appropriate analgesia should be a consideration for any ambulatory anesthetic procedure. Invasive procedures such as surgeries should be conducted once the animal is at a surgical plane and using general anesthetics; intraoperative analgesia that continues after the anesthetic recovery period should be provided to every patient.[7] Minimally invasive procedures such as biopsies and dental extractions could be performed on conscious patients with the use of local anesthetics if general anesthesia is deemed to be overly taxing for the animal subject. Such as anesthetic events involving aquatic species, where postanesthetic sedation could result in drowning. In situations when general anesthesia cannot be implemented safely, appropriate preemptive analgesia is recommended and encouraged.[7] Many anesthetics used to facilitate general anesthesia, such as propofol and inhalants, do not have an analgesic effect and should be paired with an appropriate analgesic agent. Analgesic drugs that can be used in an ambulatory scenario include opioids, antiinflammatory drugs (nonsteroidal or steroidal), and local anesthetics.[23] The American College of Veterinary Anesthesia and Analgesia provides guidelines for the recognition and treatment of pain in a variety of animal patients.[24]

Emergency Preparation

All personnel who will play the role of the anesthetists should have some basic training in anesthetic emergency management for both the veterinary patient and human personnel (see Management of Capture Drug Accidents and Human Exposure). Anesthesia and surgical personnel should have basic training in the causes of and treatments for apnea, bradycardia, tachycardia, hypothermia, and cardiopulmonary arrest. Additionally, personnel should be prepared to treat and deal with complications associated with hypoxia, hypotension, and hypoventilation.[1] Advanced monitoring techniques, including pulse oximetry, capnography, and blood pressure analysis, should be used to help identify trends; however, these techniques may not be feasible in an ambulatory setting. Although it is impossible to be completely prepared for every potential emergency, the anesthetist has an ethical responsibility to be prepared for the most common anesthetic and surgical emergencies, including respiratory distress or arrest, bradycardia arrhythmias, and cardiac arrest, hemorrhage, hypotension, and contamination of surgical sites.[1]

ANESTHETIC CONSEQUENCES AND COMPLICATIONS
Physical Trauma

When working in a field setting, there is an inherent risk of injury, including wounds and fractures associated with turbulent inductions and recoveries. Remote drug delivery equipment such as dart projectors carry a risk of injury to the animal. Such devices should only be used by trained personnel familiar with the terrain and species at hand. The anesthetist who plans to perform ambulatory anesthesia in a remote setting should be prepared for treatment or wounds, including cleaning and potentially repair.[1] Injectable antibiotics should be administered if necessary based on appropriate regulatory guidelines.

Drug Side Effects

Opioid side effects in animals can include excitement, aimless wandering, myopathy, respiratory depression, hypertension, bradycardia, muscle rigidity, and renarcotization. Renarcotization is recurrence of sedation after apparent recovery. This complication can occur when the duration of action of reversal are shorter than the opioid agonist. Chances of renarcotization could be lowered by using shorter acting opioids, additional dosing of reversals, or reducing the dose of opioid needed by adding an alpha-2 agonist or ketamine.[7]

Respiratory Depression and Hypoxia

Respiratory depression and related hypoxemia is one of the most common complications of ambulatory anesthesia. Several causative factors including immobilizing drug combinations, ventilation–perfusion mismatching poor or inappropriate positioning and airway obstruction have been noted. Clinical signs of respiratory depression and hypoxia include few, shallow, or no respirations; cyanosis (mucous membranes that are blue, gray or "muddy"); noisy breathing, wheezing, or rattling; and decreased oxygen saturation, measures of less than 85% on the pulse oximeter or a pulse oximetry reading that is trending down.[1] The recommended treatment for suspected hypoxia is to ensure appropriate positioning of the patient: the neck should be straight, tongue retracted out of the mouth, animal positing in sternal recumbency, oxygen supplementation via nasal cannulas or established airway (intubation), and artificial ventilation (Fig. 3). If there is no response to supportive treatments, it is recommended that the appropriate antagonist be given and termination of the anesthetic procedure.[1]

Temperature Dysregulation: Hyperthermia and Hypothermia

Outdoor captures carry the risk of hypothermia or hyperthermia, depending on ambient conditions. Hyperthermia is an elevated body temperature owing to failed thermoregulation that occurs when a body produces or absorbs more heat than it can dissipate owing to an increased metabolism.[7] Hyperthermia is a life-threatening condition and can be caused by overexertion and increased metabolic heat production, heat absorption from the environment, drug-induced alterations of the thermoregulatory centers, and infections. Clinical signs of hyperthermia include an elevated core or rectal temperature (>105°F in most mammals), rapid, shallow breathing (panting), rapid heart rate, and/or irregular pulse and may lead to coma or death. Treatment for hyperthermia includes actively cooling the animal and termination of the immobilization procedure with the administration of appropriate anesthetic antagonists.[7]

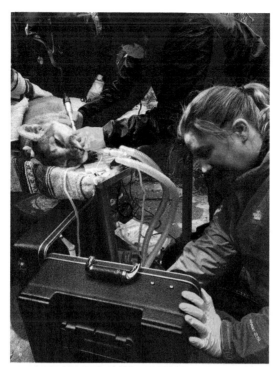

Fig. 3. An anesthetized cougar (*Puma concolor*) being ventilated with a portable anesthesia machine and monitored with battery-powered pulse oximetry and capnography.

Hypothermia is the decrease in body temperature to the point of cellular death owing in part to decreased metabolism, freezing, and/or vascular damage. Much like hyperthermia, the causes include decreased in metabolic heat production because of drug-induced alterations in metabolism or the thermoregulatory center, inadequate circulation, or a loss of body heat to the environment via evaporation, radiation, conduction, or convection.[7] Clinical signs of decreased rectal temperature (<95°F), cold extremities, shivering, and decreased heart rate and blood pressure. Treatment of hypothermia can be challenging in a remote setting; recommendations are to warm the animal via drying and warming. In most cases, a decreased metabolism will prolong the effects of immobilizing drugs and, therefore, it is recommended that the animal be warmed to near normal body temperature before the administration of any reversal agents.[7]

Exertional (Capture) Myopathy

Exertional (capture) myopathy is a condition that is associated with an adverse stressful or strenuous capture or handling.[7] The pathophysiology of this condition is complex and is linked to rapid changes in perfusion and tissue pH with exertion or restraint in which metabolic disturbances resulting from hyperlactatemia and myolysis and a rapid release of intracellular potassium. Factors such as prolonged physiologic and/or psychological stress, hyperthermia, the use of ultrapotent opioids, and hypoperfusion have been implicated in the severity of condition.[7]

Other Concerns

In addition to the concerns and complications discussed, the anesthetist should be aware that any risk and complication that can be associated with an anesthetic event in the clinical setting can also occur in a remote setting. The anesthetist should further review concerns for perianesthetic vomiting and aspiration, bloating, seizures, electrolyte imbalances, dehydration, and cardiac arrest and should have a plan in place for the treatment of these conditions.

RECOVERY CONCERNS

Considerations for the recovery of an immobilized animal after an ambulatory anesthetic event has taken place often vary depending on species, drugs used, and environment. As mentioned, it is important to have prior knowledge regarding the historic reactions of individuals of the species of interest in capture situations to better predict their recovery. In general, an animal recovering from anesthesia should not be left unobserved.[1] Ideally, the animals should be observed from a safe distance until it is able to stand and ambulate in a normal manner.

MANAGEMENT OF CAPTURE DRUG ACCIDENTS AND HUMAN EXPOSURE

There are several highly concentrated agents in production that may be considered harmful for human personnel and their accidental exposure could result in severe side effects. The most likely route of accidental exposure is inadvertent spraying in eyes, mouth, or injection via a syringe.[1] The best method for the reduction in the potential accidental human exposure is prevention.

Prevention

It is recommended that preventative training be implemented and a discussion of possible side effects of the immobilizing agents be performed before any anesthetic event. Training in appropriate equipment and drug handling, personal protective equipment requirements and cardiopulmonary resuscitation techniques should all be addressed.[1] Additionally, anesthetists should always work in pairs, with appropriate antagonists available in case of accidental exposure. Finally, the notification of local emergency personnel when ultrapotent opioids are in use is also recommended. There are several resources that are available for advanced, in-person training for the use of immobilization drugs in clinical and remote settings.[1]

SUMMARY

Field and ambulatory anesthesia is often necessary for the safe handling of exotic animals outside of the hospital setting. A thorough understanding of the specialized anesthesia equipment and handling practices for exotic animals is necessary to perform safe an effective anesthesia in the field. Clinicians are encouraged to train and familiarize themselves with remote drug delivery systems, field anesthesia monitors, and inhalant delivery systems. When practicing any type of medicine away from the hospital, proper planning and emergency preparation are critical.

REFERENCES

1. Kreeger TJ, Arnemo JM. Handbook of wildlife chemical immobilization. 4th edition. Laramie (WY): 2012.
2. Stoskopf MK, Mulcahy DM, Esler D. Evaluation of a portable automatic serum chemistry analyzer for field assessment of harlequin ducks, Historicus histrionicus. Vet Med Int 2010;2010:418596.
3. Berrie PM. Sex differences in response to phencyclidine hydrochloride in lynx. J Wildl Manage 1972;36:994–6.

4. Grubb TL, Perez Jimenez TE, Pettifer GR. Neonatal and pediatric patients. In: Grimm KA, Lamont LA, Tranquillin WJ, et al, editors. Veterinary anesthesia and analgesia. 5th edition. Ames (IA): John Wiley & Sons, Inc; 2015. p. 983–7.

5. Grubb TL, Perez Jimenez TE, Pettifer GR. Senior and geriatric patients. In: Grimm KA, Lamont LA, Tranquillin WJ, et al, editors. Veterinary anesthesia and analgesia. 5th edition. Ames (IA): John Wiley & Sons, Inc; 2015. p. 988–92.

6. Caulkett NA, Arnemo JM. Comparative anesthesia and analgesia of zoo animals. In: Grimm KA, Lamont LA, Tranquillin WJ, et al, editors. Veterinary anesthesia and analgesia. 5th edition. Ames (IA): John Wiley & Sons, Inc; 2015. p. 764–76.

7. Chinnadurai SK, Strahl-Heldreth D, Fiorello CV, et al. Best-practice guidelines for field-based surgery and anesthesia of free-ranging wildlife. I. Anesthesia and analgesia. J Wildl Dis 2016;52(2s):S14–27.

8. Hawkins MG, Barron H, Speer BL, et al. Birds. In: Carpenter JW, editor. Exotic animal formulary. 4th edition. St Louis (MO): Elsevier Saunders; 2013. p. 183–437.

9. Cooper JE, Appendix IX. Medicines and other agents used in treatment, including emergency anaesthesia kit and avian resuscitation protocol. In: Cooper JE, editor. Birds of prey: health and disease. 3rd edition. Ames (IO): Blackwell Publishing, Iowa State Press; 2002. p. 271–7.

10. Padilla LR, Ko JC. Nondomestic suids. In: West G, Heard D, Caulkett N, editors. Zoo animal and wildlife immobilization and anesthesia. 2nd edition. Ames (MO): Wiley Blackwell; 2014. p. 773–85.

11. Masters N. Primates. In: Meredith A, Johnson-Delaney C, editors. BSAVA manual of exotic pets. 5th edition. Quedgeley (England): British Small Animal Veterinary Association; 2010. p. 148–66.

12. Cerveny S, Sleeman J. Great apes. In: West G, Heard D, Caulkett N, editors. Zoo animal and wild-life immobilization and anesthesia. 2nd edition. Ames (MO): John Wiley & Sons; 2014. p. 573–84.

13. Brainard B, Darrow EJ. Sedation and anesthesia in the great apes—an overview. Proc Annu Conf Am Assoc Zoo Vet 2013;26–35.

14. Cattet MR, Caulkett NA, Wilson C, et al. Intranasal administration of xylazine to help reduce stress in elk captured by net gun. J Wildl Dis 2004;40:562–5.

15. Lacoste L, Bouquet S, Ingrand P, et al. Intranasal midazolam in piglets: pharmacodynamics (0.2 vs 0.4 mg/kg) and pharmacokinetics (0.4mg/kg) with bioavailability determination. Lab Anim 2000;34:29–35.

16. Araghi M, Azizi S, Vesal N, et al. Evaluation of the sedative effects of diazepam, midazolam, and xylazine after intranasal administration in juvenile ostriches (*Struthio camelus*). J Avian Med Surg 2016;30:221–6.

17. Mylniczenko ND, Neiffer DL, Clauss TM. Bony fish (lungfish, sturgeon, and teleosts). In: West G, Heard D, Caulkett N, editors. Zoo animal and wildlife immobilization and anesthesia. 2nd edition. Ames (IA): John Wiley & Sons, Inc; 2014. p. 209–60.

18. Neiffer DL, Stamper MA. Fish Sedation, anesthesia, analgesia, and euthanasia: considerations, methods, and types of drugs. ILAR J 2009;50(4):343–60.

19. Mosley CI, Mosley CA. Comparative anesthesia and analgesia of reptiles, amphibians, and fishes. In: Grimm KA, Lamont LA, Tranquillin WJ, et al, editors. Veterinary anesthesia and analgesia. 5th edition. Ames (IA): John Wiley & Sons, Inc; 2015. p. 784–99.

20. Stetter MD. Fish and amphibian anesthesia. Vet Clin North Am Exot Anim Pract 2001;4:69–82.

21. International Air Transport Association. IATA dangerous goods regulations. 54th edition. Montreal (Canada): International Air Transport Association; 2013.

22. Branson K. Injectable and alternative anesthetic techniques. In: Thurmon J, Tranquilli W, Grimm K, editors. Veterinary anesthesia and analgesia. 4th edition. Ames (IA): Blackwell; 2007. p. 273–99.

23. Whiteside DP. Analgesia. In: West G, Heard D, Caulkett N, editors. Zoo animal and wildlife immobilization and anesthesia. 2nd edition. Ames (IA): John Wiley & Sons, Inc; 2014. p. 83–108.

24. American College of Veterinary Anesthesia and Analgesia (ACVAA). American College of Veterinary Anesthesiologists' position paper on the treatment of pain in animals. 2006. Available at: http://acvaa.org/docs/Pain_Treatment. Accessed March 1, 2018.

Aquatic Ambulatory Practice

Jessie Sanders, DVM, CertAqV

KEYWORDS

- Mobile • Ambulatory • Aquarium • Tank • Pond • Fish • Koi • Goldfish

KEY POINTS

- Ambulatory aquatic animal veterinary practice incorporates environmental assessments into clinical cases.
- Most diagnostics and procedures can be performed on aquatic patients in an ambulatory setting.
- Specific equipment for catching patients in an efficient and timely manner is required for the ambulatory practitioner.
- Treatment options must be considered with the client's involvement, comfort, and understanding.

INTRODUCTION

Aquatic ambulatory practice has the benefit of bringing veterinarians tank or pond side, allowing for a thorough evaluation of a patient's aquatic environment. Many larger fish, such as koi and sturgeon, are difficult to transport, thereby making an ambulatory component essential to any aquatic animal veterinary practice. The most important skill of the ambulatory practitioner is to be able to catch your intended patient quickly and efficiently to reduce stress and comorbidity. This can be accomplished with skill, patience, and nets of many sizes and purposes. Many of the common aquatic diagnostic techniques can be used pond or tank side. Coordination with another veterinary practice can extend the availability of veterinary services.

What Does It Take to Make an Ambulatory Aquatics Practice?

Establishing an ambulatory aquatic practice is relatively simple compared with a conventional small or large animal private practice. With its ambulatory nature, most practitioners will be able to work independently with a few additional tools. It is highly recommended that a Web site be created specific for the practice or add a page to your existing clinic Web site. Because of its novel nature, potential clients will rely on your Web site and clinic referrals to find your services.

Disclosure: The author has nothing to disclose.
Aquatic Veterinary Services, 440 Airport Boulevard, Watsonville, CA 95076, USA
E-mail addresses: vet@cafishvet.com; cafishvet@gmail.com

Vet Clin Exot Anim 21 (2018) 609–622
https://doi.org/10.1016/j.cvex.2018.05.003
1094-9194/18/© 2018 Elsevier Inc. All rights reserved.

Staffing

Additional staffing is at the discretion of the practitioner. If a clinic is already established, all of your staffing for fielding calls and triaging will be in place. Make sure staff is aware of what information to collect from callers (**Box 1**). If practicing without any support staff, an answering service may be hired to collect the same set of information, or have potential clients fill out an online form. The complete summary can be e-mailed or faxed to the operations base. Set up a message on your work phone directing clients how to best contact you.

Pricing and Fee Structure

Pricing is at the discretion of the practitioner; however, keep in mind that this is a highly specialized, *ambulatory* practice. Providing service that is hard to find and on location should be considered a premium. There is a strong urge to underprice when getting started.

Fee structure can be set up as an hourly, à la carte, or package option. Hourly fees will include travel from the home base. À la carte and package options need to have a separate item for travel, which can be done by the minute or mile. The travel range of the veterinary practitioner will influence the scope of clients, so bear this in mind when setting your fee structure. Package options can include water quality testing and a few fish examinations under sedation, including capture. All treatments with this option can be à la carte. Re-check fees are usually at lower cost than first-time clients.

Equipment

Much of the veterinary equipment is the same as for small/large animal practice (eg, needles, syringes, drugs); however, an aquatic practitioner will require an assortment of nets and buckets to accommodate a wide range of fish sizes (1 inch to 24+ inches). Portable scales will be necessary to obtain fish weights and need to be water-resistant. A water quality test kit and microscope are suggested as part of a mobile

---

Box 1
Example of form for answering service to fill out and fax to our office

Date/Time:

Initials:

Type of call: Routine/Emergency/Question/Medication Request

Primary issue:

Name:

Phone:

E-mail:

Type of fish:

How many fish affected:

Duration of symptoms:

How big is the pond:

Last water change:

How much water was changed:

setup, but can be performed at the home base. Although not necessary, a portable centrifuge, suction unit, and ultrasound are useful to have. Make sure to bring lots of towels for keeping hands dry and cleaning up spills in a client's home (**Figs. 1–8**).

In addition to the preceding items, there are other suggested items that may be helpful to carry (**Box 2**).

As with all veterinary practice, sanitation and cleaning of equipment must occur between client visits. Multiple sets of equipment are beneficial for practitioners with many days of multiple patients. There are many appropriate aquatic sanitation protocols available.[1] Chlorine bleach of any kind is toxic to fish and must be deactivated before using in another pond. Virkon is the only drug approved for use in commercial aquaculture. Other possible disinfectants include Clorox, Roccal-D, Lysol, ethyl alcohol, and glutaraldehyde.[2]

TYPES OF CLIENTS (DEMOGRAPHICS)

- Outdoor ponds
- Indoor tanks
- Aquaculture
- Small-scale public aquaria

A variety of clients may benefit from an ambulatory aquatic animal practice. The standard indoor fish tank hobbyist is most capable of transporting small fish to a traditional hospital, but larger fish and systems will need on-site assistance. Clients uncomfortable with transporting critically ill or injured fish are the most grateful for ambulatory practice. Outdoor koi pond keepers are the most common clients requiring on-site visits. Koi living in large outdoor ponds can be difficult to catch by owners and can often have more than one fish affected. The wide variety of pond setups and mixing of species can complicate any aquatic disease. Many koi owners

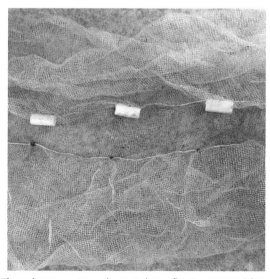

Fig. 1. Seine net. These large, rectangular nets have floats on one side and weights on the other. Starting from one side of a large pond, these nets are slowly brought across to cordon the fish into a smaller, more manageable area.

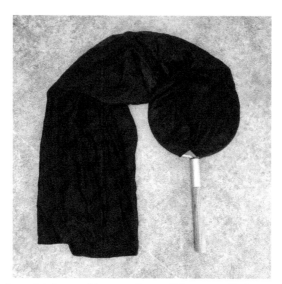

Fig. 2. Sock net. Essential for catching any larger fish, especially koi, these permeable or nonpermeable soft nets are fabric tubes open at both ends. The soft material keeps large fish from damage while transporting between pond and examination tub. Permeable varieties allow water to pass through and should be used with any treated water. Nonpermeable sock nets are used for transport between nontreated systems.

are often underprepared for basic problems, so veterinarians will need to understand and resolve husbandry issues.

Among the koi hobbyists are koi show keepers. These clients tend to have more expensive fish and will have certain aesthetic requirements. Koi show winners can

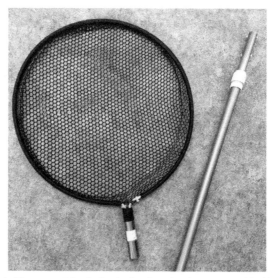

Fig. 3. Herding net. Also a must for koi veterinarians is a large, round koi-herding net. These nets are not intended to be used for transport out of the water, but rather for moving koi to an area where a sock net can be used. They come in very large varieties (18–36 inches) but can be difficult to maneuver. A detachable handle is recommended for easier transport.

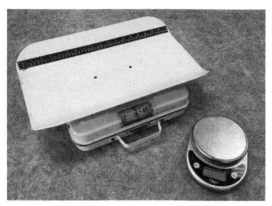

Fig. 4. A portable scale for large and small fish is critical for the ambulatory practitioner.

go for several thousands of dollars, so considerable care must be taken with their treatment and handling. A little knowledge about the traditional varieties of koi and how shows operate is of great benefit to the aquatic practitioner.

Aquaculture farms are required to have face-to-face interaction with a veterinarian to validate any certificates of veterinary inspection or Veterinary Feed Directive (VFD). This will satisfy the veterinarian-client-patient relationship. The frequency of these visits will vary by state, but all require an on-site veterinary inspection. These clients require ambulatory veterinary service to fully function.

Small-scale public aquaria do not require a full-time veterinarian. They may require veterinary assistance on a monthly or quarterly basis, or only as an animal becomes ill.

EVALUATION OF ENVIRONMENT (HISTORY TO INCLUDE)

A significant advantage to ambulatory practice is on-site evaluation of the patient's environment. It is recommended that all visits include a walkthrough of equipment

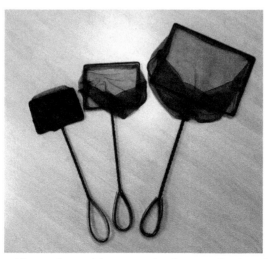

Fig. 5. Capture nets. All aquatic practitioners need to have a collection of nets for small fish and other aquatic animals. Nets with a finer weave are recommended because they snag less on fin rays.

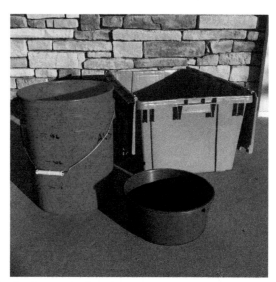

Fig. 6. Examination buckets and tubs will vary by the size of the patient. It is recommended that a variety is kept from a 5-L painter's pail to 60-L file box. Five-gallon buckets will also work well for many sizes of fish and are necessary to fill larger containers. A sump pump can be used to fill and empty buckets that are too heavy for the practitioner.

with the owner or system caretaker. The items listed in **Box 3** should be addressed and identified.

Systems will vary widely, especially with koi ponds. Identifying the individual components at the start of an appointment will allow you to make suggestions for changes

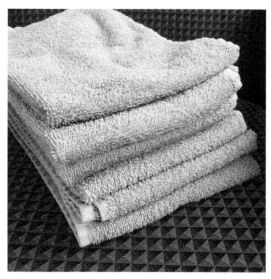

Fig. 7. In working with aquatic patients, water is inevitable. Have plenty of towels on hand to keep your hands dry when performing diagnostics and mopping up any water spilled in a client's home.

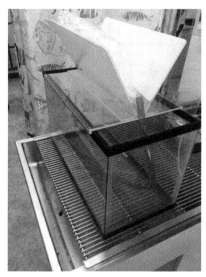

Fig. 8. Mobile surgical table set up over 10-gallon aquarium tank. Acrylic V-shape can be tailored to many different fish shapes and sizes. It can be flipped over to work with fish on their sides. A small aquarium pump brings water up from the reservoir underneath.

after diagnosing the chief complaint. All fish case histories must include environmental management practices and routines. Many common diseases in ambulatory veterinary practice are secondary to poor husbandry.[3,4] The environment and its management can significantly impact fish health.

When evaluating the environment, a visual inspection of animals that are not considered sick by the client needs to be performed. Client ability on identification of sick aquatic animals varies widely and it is up to the visiting veterinarian to assess the health of all animals in the environment (**Fig. 9**).

HANDLING, CAPTURE, AND TRANSPORT

Correct handling of aquatic patients is a primary concern during an ambulatory visit. Most smaller fish can be handled without sedation, whereas larger koi will need sedation to limit injury to themselves. New techniques are emerging for training fish for cooperative routine diagnostic procedures.[5] Aquaculture visits need to be coordinated with staff to procure appropriate age and size of fish before arrival or during visit.

Box 2
Suggested items

Foldable table for setting up equipment

Head lamp for darker environments

Rain/sun protection for equipment

Fish transport bags and rubber bands with additional oxygen for potentially long transports

Knee protection: kneepads or kneeling boards

Portable suction and centrifuge

Small cooler for potential sample transport

Box 3
Life Support Systems to assess

Mechanical filtration (eg, sponges, pads, settling tank)

Biological filtration (eg, beads, bio balls, matting, sponges)

Drainage (eg, skimmer, bottom drain)

System flow-through

Aeration (waterfalls or air stones)

UV and other specialized filtration

If you will be euthanizing patients for aquaculture sampling, consider a method of euthanasia that allows the animals to be consumed after sampling.

Before starting capture, note which fish need to be caught. If no disease processes or fish specified by the client are present, a random sampling will suffice. It is recommended at least 3 fish in each system be sampled at minimum. Presumably healthy individuals should be caught and examined before sick and injured fish.

When catching fish, proceed in a calm and planned method to minimize stress levels. Capture and handling-related stress can significantly impact fish health.[6–8] If possible, remove any obstructions or hiding places, such as décor or cave coverings. Use multiple nets if necessary to herd animals to a smaller, more manageable area. It will take time to build up the appropriate net handling and coordination. Less-practiced veterinarians may work best using a herding net in each hand to sandwich the intended target. Having clients or additional staff assist in capture may hinder capture efforts more than help if they are unfamiliar with the practice.

Always time how long it takes to capture a fish. This is the time your net enters the water until the fish is transferred to the examination tub. Stress due to capture can cause an increase in disease processes after the veterinary visit.[9] Therefore, the shortest time to capture will result in the lowest chance of disease. If capture is unsuccessful after 10 minutes, the technique needs to be reassessed and possibly halted for the time being. If a second attempt is to be made, consider additional equipment or personnel.

Some fish in need of further nursing care need to be moved to a more appropriate environment for proper healing. This may be more important in ponds or tanks with poor water quality, overcrowding, seasonal changes, and other factors that are out of the veterinarian's control. A fish may be able to remain in its original environment if the owner is willing to work on improving the system, including rehoming fish, building a quarantine system, or improving maintenance protocols. As with capture, proper transport techniques are essential.[10] Proper acclimation will also need to occur when the fish reaches the destination. If the veterinarian is not present during these events, clear, written instructions need to be given to both the shipper and receiver.

Hospitalization is up to the practitioner. Holding smaller fish, such as bettas, small tropicals, and goldfish can be accomplished in an indoor tank setup at the hospital or practitioner's home. This small setup is done for little space and cost, but allows the fish to receive more direct treatments when isolated. The space to hold larger fish, such as koi, requires a larger footprint and may be several thousand gallons. If the practitioner has the space, a large, heated koi quarantine tub can be very useful. If the practitioner lacks the space to do this, the practitioner may rent a temporary tub to owners with an all-in-one filter option. Some fish owners are very reluctant to set up another separate quarantine system. Take the time to educate them on how a proper quarantine system is a great asset for sick, injured, or new fish.[11]

Client: _____

Date: _____

Primary complaint:

History:

Water Quality:

Ammonia: _____ mg/L   Nitrite: _____ mg/L   Nitrate: _____ mg/L

pH: _____   Alkalinity: _____ mg/L   Hardness: _____ mg/L

Oxygen: _____ mg/L   Temperature: _____ F

Differentials:

Plan to correct:

Fish Physicals:

Fish 1: _____

Skin   Gills   Body   Etc

Fish 2: _____

Skin   Gills   Body   Etc

Fish 3: _____

Skin   Gills   Body   Etc

Findings:

Treatment Plan:

Signature

Fig. 9. Visit form used during appointment to capture information. (*Courtesy of* Aquatic Veterinary Services, Soquel, CA; with permission.)

DIAGNOSTICS

A complete guide to diagnostic testing in fish can be found in the published literature.[12] **Table 1** is a list of diagnostics that must be completed on-site versus those that can be completed at the office or laboratory.[13–15] All samples collected in the field

Table 1	
Diagnostics	
On-Site	**Hospital/Laboratory**
Water quality parameter testing	Blood processing
Skin mucus, fin and bill biopsy, and analysis	Stained cytology processing
Histopathology samples on euthanasia	Histopathology
Cytology collection	Viral, bacterial, and fungal processing
Blood collection	Radiographs/ultrasound
Radiographs/ultrasound	

Data from Refs.[13–15]

need to be transported correctly, so traveling with a small cooler is highly recommended. Ice and other coolants can be obtained from any grocery or drug store.

Some practitioners will not have readily available access to more advanced diagnostics, such as radiographs and ultrasound. It is recommended to coordinate these tests with a local small animal hospital. Protection of equipment from water with plastic sheeting and towels may be necessary and should be considered before use. Communicate with hospital staff that the aquatic veterinarian will be present for all procedures and perform necessary sedation and positioning if necessary. Most small animal hospitals will have never examined a fish and may be reluctant/hesitant to agree if they assume the fish will simply be dropped off. Assure on-site staff they are responsible only for working the equipment, the ambulatory aquatic practitioner will handle sedation and placement and will protect the equipment from getting wet.

Diagnostics performed on dead specimens will not be of use unless the fish has died while on-site or recently deceased and properly refrigerated. Fish that die overnight or the day before the visit are of little diagnostic value. Dead fish decompose too rapidly and unless they are found just after they die, there is no viable tissue that can be tested.

TREATMENT OPTIONS AND FOLLOW-UP CARE

Following diagnosis, treatment options need to be discussed with the client. All have benefits and difficulties depending on the client and the client's comfort level.[16–18]

Immersion-Based Treatment

One of the most common treatment methods, this option requires proper client education about how the system needs to be handled throughout the duration of treatment. Depending on the chemicals or drugs used, this type of treatment can significantly impact biological filtration function. Once the treatment has been administered, it is up to the practitioner to allow clients to perform follow-up treatments or have them administered by the veterinarian. Proper disposal of treated water and any excess chemicals needs to be discussed with clients before departure.

Feed-Based Treatment

After prescribing and manufacturing, information about its storage, use, and dissemination needs to be discussed with the client. However, this is a simple treatment for clients to perform without the supervision of a veterinarian. It can be a more expensive treatment than immersion-based, but is guaranteed not to affect the biological filtration. This is especially significant with aquaculture producers and VFDs. They will have specific recommendations, as the species, life stage, and disease requiring treatment and multiple VFDs may be necessary.

Injectable Treatment

This method of treatment requires the veterinarian administer all treatments and follow-ups. It is usually the most expensive method of treatment, given that the veterinarian's time is required and most stressful because the fish will need to be handled further. It is a highly effective treatment and will not harm the biological filtration. This method should be first considered in areas that have severe water restrictions.

Surgical Treatment

Surgical procedures may be performed during ambulatory visits. Short-duration external surgeries, such as cutaneous tumor removals, cryotherapy, or enucleations are safe to perform in an appropriate environment with good water quality.[19–22] More advanced surgical procedures, such as exploratory coelomic surgery, are better to take place in more sterile settings but can be performed on-site.[23] Mobile surgery setups can be fabricated for use in ambulatory service if necessary. If a client's pond is not adequate for healing, the fish may need to be relocated and brought back after they are completely healed. As discussed previously, it is up to the practitioner's time and space allocation if they are able to offer hospitalization.

CASE EXAMPLES
Koi Pond with Ectoparasites

A common koi case occurs in the spring and early summer. An owner will call saying the fish are lethargic, clamped fins, decreased appetites, and/or reddening of the skin on pale-colored fish. On inspection of the pond, water quality parameters, and physical examination, external parasites are noted in the skin mucus and/or gills. Coming out of colder temperatures, these parasites take advantage of a fish's weakened immune system to cause severe skin irritation, respiratory distress, and secondary bruising. This is also common after the addition of new, unquarantined fish. Parasite infections can be exacerbated by poor water quality. After the parasite has been diagnosed, proper treatment options can be discussed with the clients.

Upside-Down Fancy Goldfish

Fancy goldfish have been bred for outward appearance and not internal function and form. Fancy goldfish are prone to buoyancy disorders, both positive and negative. As part of any good aquatic veterinary examination, test the water parameters first, for some buoyancy disorders are caused by poor water quality alone.[24] Provided these are within optimal parameters, inquire after the fish's diet. Goldfish are physostomous, with a duct between their esophagus and swim bladder. Switching the diet may be able to correct the disorder. Radiographs may be required to evaluate the shape and positioning of the swim bladder. Goldfish with polycystic kidney disease (PKD) may have reduced or repositioned swim bladders affecting buoyancy. PKD can be diagnosed by aspirate or ultrasound. Some fancy goldfish will have permanent buoyancy disorders and must be kept with extra care.

Koi with Swollen Coelom

Koi with a swollen coelom or distended belly are common in the warmer summer months during spawning season. In spring and late summer, the swelling is caused by egg maturation and will spawn when appropriate.[25] Egg retention is a concern in koi. Other times, the enlargement is caused by an internal neoplasia. It may be a benign neoplasia, in the form of a cyst, or a solid, tissue neoplasia. Diagnosis can be made using cytology or ultrasound. Treatments vary from a simple suction to open coelomic surgery.

"Old Tank" and "New Tank" Syndromes

Common with inexperienced hobbyists, old tank syndrome (OTS) and new tank syndrome (NTS) are caused by inappropriate maintenance causing many secondary fish diseases, including bacterial and fungal infections. This syndrome also can occur in ponds. OTS is characterized by a depletion of the available buffers in solution causing a slow pH decrease. The decrease in pH leads to a deactivation of the biological filtration and an increase in ammonia levels. This syndrome can be corrected by doing many small water changes to add buffers and reduce the ammonia.

NTS occurs in recently established systems in which the biological filtration has yet to be established. It also can occur in systems in which the filtration is cleaned too aggressively. This leads to an ammonia spike that can lead to death and secondary disease. A nitrite spike can follow afterward, as the bacterial colonies are established. Bacterial colonies will be established in approximately 4 to 6 weeks. Water changes and decreasing stocking density will help in preventing secondary signs.

TRAINING AND FURTHER LEARNING

Additional support for aquatic practitioners can be obtained through networking with other aquatic professionals (**Table 2**). Education on aquatic animal health and veterinary skills can be gained through one of the aquatic veterinary programs (**Table 3**). Professional publications and conference proceedings also can be found online at VIN.com.

TIPS AND TRICKS

- When considering pricing for ambulatory aquatic service, take into consideration how few specialties across human and veterinary medicine provide at-home services. An ambulatory specialty veterinary service is a very beneficial and unique service and must be priced accordingly. Consider offering different pricing structures for large ponds versus indoor tanks versus aquaculture assessments.
- It takes time to build up proper fish-catching skills. New practitioners should know how to use all types of nets and use multiple nets at once to ensure a quick and efficient capture. If possible, practice using different nets in a pool or tub to get a sense of how they handle under the pressure of the water. It is always best to move slowly when working with fish, so they do not dart away and possibly hurt themselves running into an obstacle.
- One veterinarian's method of catching koi: In larger ponds, start by using a seine net to herd the fish to a smaller area. Mind the sides of the net; this is where most fish will slip through. If you have an assistant, have the assistant hold one end of the net flush against the side of the pond, then pull the loose side in a sweeping

Table 2 Aquatic veterinary organizations		
American Association of Fish Veterinarians	AAFV	https://fishvets.org
World Aquatic Veterinary Medical Association	WAVMA	https://wavma.org
International Association of Aquatic Animal Medicine	IAAAM	https://iaaam.org

Table 3	
Aquatic educational opportunities	
AQUAVET	https://www2.vet.cornell.edu/education/other-educational-opportunities/aquavet
MARVET	http://www.marvet.org/
SeaVet	http://www.conference.ifas.ufl.edu/seavet/index.html

motion around the entire perimeter of the pond. Use the large, round herd net to guide your intended patient to the surface. Keep in mind that fish may try to jump over your net when they get close to the surface. Angle the herd net above the water line to prevent them from escaping. The herd net also can be used to pin a fish against the side of the pond. Use the sock net to capture the fish, moving head to tail and holding the 2 ends in both hands. Keep the net spread wide when moving the fish from the pond to examination tub. When your examination is complete, move the sedated fish back to the pond. Use the large herd net to gently place the fish in a well-aerated area.

- Develop your own forms to take down all information during an ambulatory visit, including all equipment and environmental factors. Make sure to include room for a small sketch of the pond or take a picture if the client allows.
- When booking appointments to see a fish, make sure to ask the dimensions of the pond. The size of the pond will determine what equipment you need to bring. Other information to collection before making a visit is the species, number of fish affected, the onset of the symptoms, and what treatments the client has already attempted.
- If possible, have the owner send you pictures or videos over e-mail with their concerns before their appointment. Some fish behaviors and diseases can be hard to verbalize and are easier to understand through visual methods.

SUMMARY

The ability to practice effective ambulatory aquatic veterinary medicine is an attainable goal for any veterinary practitioner. In addition to new equipment, new skills must be developed and practiced frequently to deliver timely results. Diagnostics and treatments proceed similarly to any aquatic practitioner with some requiring follow-up. Keep in mind that an ambulatory aquatic animal veterinarian is a unique specialty and should be priced accordingly. Ambulatory practice is a great benefit to all fish keepers with large fish or critically sick or injured pets.

REFERENCES

1. Mainous ME, Smith SA. Efficacy of common disinfectants against *Mycobacterium marinum*. J Aqua Anim Health 2005;17:284–8.
2. Mainous ME, Smith SA, Kuhn DD. Effect of common aquaculture chemicals against *Edwardsiella ictaluri*. J Aqua Anim Health 2011;22(4):224–8.
3. Cecil TR. Husbandry and husbandry-related diseases of ornamental fish. Vet Clin North Am Exot Anim Pract 1999;2(1):1–18.
4. Roberts H, Palmeiro BS. Toxicology of aquarium fish. Vet Clin North Am Exot Anim Pract 2008;11(2):359–74.
5. Corwin AL. Training fish and aquatic invertebrates for husbandry and medical behaviors. Vet Clin North Am Exot Anim Pract 2012;15(3):455–67.

6. Harmon TS. Methods for reducing stressors and maintaining water quality associated with live fish transport in tanks: a review of the basics. Rev Aquaculture 2009;1:58–66.

7. Maule AG, Schreck CB, Samual BC, et al. Physiological effects of collecting and transporting emigrating juvenile chinook salmon past dams on the Columbia River. Trans Am Fish Soc 1988;117:245–61.

8. Robertson L, Thomas P, Arnold CR. Plasma cortisol and secondary stress responses of cultured red drum (*Scianenops ocellatus*) to several transportation procedures. Aquaculture 1988;68:115–30.

9. Noga EJ, Botts S, Yang MS, et al. Acute stress causes skin ulceration in striped bass and hybrid bass (*Morone*). Vet Pathol 1998;35:102–7.

10. Yeager DM, Van Tassel JE, Wooley CM. Collection, transportation, and handling of striped bass brood stock. In: Harrell RM, Kerby JH, Monton RV, editors. Culture and propagation of striped bass and its hybrids. Bethesda (MD): American Fisheries Society; 1990. p. 39–42.

11. Arthur JR, Bondad-Reantaso MG, Subasinghe RP. Procedures for the quarantine of live aquatic animals: a manual. FAO Fisheries Technical Paper 502. 2008.

12. Reavill DR. Common diagnostic and clinical techniques for fish. Vet Clin North Am Exot Anim Pract 2006;9:223–35.

13. Roberts HE, Palmeiro B, Weber ES III. Bacterial and parasitic diseases of pet fish. Vet Clin North Am Exot Anim Pract 2009;12(3):609–38.

14. Saint-Erne N. Diagnostic techniques and treatments for internal disorders of koi (*Cyprinus carpio*). Vet Clin North Am Exot Anim Pract 2010;13(3):333–47.

15. Groff JM, Zinkl JG. Hematology and clinical chemistry of cyprinid fish: common carp and goldfish. Vet Clin North Am Exot Anim Pract 1999;2(3):741–76.

16. Petty BD, Francis-Flloyd R. Pet fish care and husbandry. Vet Clin North Am Exot Anim Pract 2004;7:397–419.

17. Noga EJ. Fish disease: diagnosis and treatment. 2nd edition. Hoboken (NJ): Wiley-Blackwell; 2011.

18. Mashima TY, Lewbart GA. Pet fish formulary. Vet Clin North Am Exot Anim Pract 2000;3(1):117–30.

19. Roberts HE. Fundamentals of ornamental fish health. Hoboken (NJ): Wiley-Blackwell; 2010.

20. Harms CA, Lewbart GA. Surgery in fish. Vet Clin North Am Exot Anim Pract 2000; 3(3):759–74.

21. Vergneau-Grosset C, Nadeay ME, Groff JM. Fish oncology: diseases, diagnostics, and therapeutics. Vet Clin North Am Exot Anim Pract 2017;20(1):21–56.

22. Groff JM. Neoplasia in fishes. Vet Clin North Am Exot Anim Pract 2004;7(3): 705–56.

23. Wildgoose WH. Fish surgery: an overview. Fish Vet J 2000;5:22–36.

24. Wildgoose WH. Buoyancy disorders of ornamental fish: a review of cases seen in veterinary practice. Fish Vet J 2007;9:22–37.

25. Yanong RPE, Martinez C, Watson CA. Use of ovaprim in ornamental fish aquaculture. University of Florida: IFAS Extension; 2009. FA161. Available at: http://edis.ifas.ufl.edu/fa161.

Reptilian and Amphibian Ambulatory Practice
Challenges and Opportunities

Bradley J. Waffa, MSPH, DVM[a],*, Richard S. Funk, MA, DVM[b,c]

KEYWORDS

- Amphibian • Reptilian • Herpetological medicine • Reptiles • Amphibians
- Ambulatory veterinary medicine • Mobile veterinary practice

KEY POINTS

- Herpetoculture has exploded in popularity since the 1980s and has evolved dramatically since. Veterinarians have kept pace clinically, but should also consider other ways to meet the needs of this unique and changing patient demographic.
- An ambulatory visit represents a nontraditional "farm call," so that population health can be assessed; modern herpetoculture lends itself well to this approach.
- Ambulatory practice offers unique clinical, economic, psychological, and logistical benefits to veterinarians and owners of reptilian and amphibian patients.
- Safety, preparedness, scheduling, and billing can be hurdles for the reptilian and amphibian ambulatory practitioner, but they bring opportunities too.
- Although some services are offered more effectively through a standing facility, many procedures on reptiles and amphibians can be performed on an ambulatory basis.

INTRODUCTION

Herpetoculture, defined here as the collection and propagation of live reptiles and amphibians in captivity, has evolved tremendously over the past few decades. Perhaps the most satisfying change observed by veterinarians has been a slow paradigm shift in the public away from the notion that reptiles and amphibians are disposable pets.[1] To the contrary, many are long-lived, intelligent, and well-suited to healthy captive lifestyles with proper care, so it is not surprising that there has been a massive increase in their popularity, and in captive breeding efforts by private keepers. These efforts, combined with many advances in reptile and amphibian medicine and surgery, including the establishment of the Association of Reptilian and Amphibian Veterinarians

Disclosure: The authors have nothing to disclose.
[a] Gentle Care Animal Hospital, 100 Kumar Court, Raleigh, NC 27606, USA; [b] Veterinary Clinical Sciences, College of Veterinary Medicine, Midwestern University, 19555 N 59th Avenue, Glendale, AZ 85308, USA; [c] Richard Funk Veterinary Services LLC, 7718 E Palm Lane, Mesa, AZ 85207, USA
* Corresponding author.
E-mail address: bjwaffa@ncsu.edu

(ARAV) in 1990 and a dedicated board specialty in reptile and amphibian practice through the American Board of Veterinary Practitioners (ABVP) in 2010, have helped elevate herptiles from second-class pets to fixtures in elaborate collections that are growing and thriving.

Likely the most dramatic, measurable shift since the 1980s has been a trend toward larger and more diverse private herpetological collections. A practice once restricted to zoologic and museum collections is now frequently encountered in the home or as part of a small business. In 2009, there were an estimated 4.7 million US households that owned 13.6 million reptile pets, and the years prior, between 1994 and 2008, saw 68% growth in the number of those households.[2] Herpetoculture has undoubtedly continued its exponential growth in the decade since.

Although there are certainly clients that casually keep only one or a few individual reptiles or amphibians, it is increasingly common to find private keepers who view their animals as a collection of scientifically or economically important "specimens" rather than strictly as pets[3] (**Fig. 1**). For keepers with these types of collections, the traditional small animal practice model may be unaccommodating at best, and sometimes even objectionable, with some keepers preferring to forego veterinary care rather than spend time and money with a hospital they feel is incapable of meeting their needs. As herpetoculture continues to grow in popularity, and as keeping practices evolve, veterinarians must remain flexible to meet the changing needs of this patient population and the clients who tend it. Offering ambulatory services represents an innovative way for practitioners to meet these needs and evolve alongside this growing demographic.

Although offering ambulatory service may revolutionize the way one practices medicine, ambulatory practice for exotics is not a novel concept. D. Johnson, DVM, Dipl. ABVP (ECM), noted (written communication, December 2017) that some of the very first exotics-exclusive practices more than 20 years ago actually began as ambulatory practices. With minimal infrastructure and overhead, this form of practice was less expensive to operate compared with brick-and-mortar practices. Indeed, one of the authors (RSF) started an exclusively exotics ambulatory practice in Florida in 1990, with more than 90% of the patients being reptiles and amphibians. For more

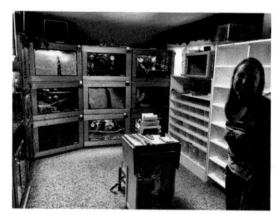

Fig. 1. It is increasingly common for private keepers of reptiles and amphibians to maintain large, elaborate collections. This herpetoculturist keeps an exquisite collection of captive-bred green tree pythons (*Morelia viridis*) in her home. (*Courtesy of* Bradley J. Waffa, MSPH, DVM, Raleigh, NC.)

information on this topic, see Todd Driggers' article, "Incorporating/Integrating Exotic Ambulatory Medicine into a Brick and Mortar Practice," elsewhere in this issue.

Historically speaking, however, ambulatory practices have been exceptions to the rule for most herpetoculturists. Traditionally, reptile owners faced with a sick animal were forced, by circumstance, to contact a local veterinary hospital to schedule an outpatient examination. Before the late 1980s, this was almost always a general practitioner, and if a client was lucky, it was one with a modicum of interest in herptiles. This has changed, as more veterinarians have declared a special interest, joined professional organizations like the ARAV, enrolled in continuing education and other postgraduate training, or even earned board certification as a reptile and amphibian specialist.

Despite these professional developments, many practitioners maintain a small animal business model in which pets are seen in the clinic on a primarily outpatient basis and where the client is charged per pet for care. This works well for practices that only occasionally see reptile or amphibian patients and for clients who keep a single or small number of these pets. But for clients with larger collections, this model is impractical. A $60 outpatient wellness examination fee may seem reasonable to the client with a single pet tortoise, but it will be rightfully rejected by a client with a collection of fifty snakes that appear outwardly healthy.

Failing to accommodate these clients' unique needs may deter them from establishing a veterinary relationship at all, because veterinarians may be perceived as inaccessibly expensive at best, or appearing exclusive at worst. At a time when trust in the veterinary profession is at a historical low, the importance of earning and maintaining client trust cannot be overstated.[4] Many herp practitioners recommend annual examinations, a wellness practice that has been well-established in dogs and cats by the American Animal Health Association and the American Veterinary Medical Association.[5,6] This recommendation, however, has been met with almost universally poor compliance from clients with large collections, likely due in part to financial and logistical impracticality. It does not have to be this way.

DISCUSSION
Advantages of Ambulatory Practice

Fortunately, where the small animal private practice model falls short of meeting the needs of many modern herpetoculturists, reptile and amphibian practitioners need not reinvent the wheel. Veterinarians have been servicing a surprisingly similar patient population for as long as our profession has existed: agricultural livestock in a production setting. Although there are obviously stark biological differences between these groups of animals, a ball python obviously shares little in common with a Holstein cow, the clients who manage them actually share many of the same concerns: economy of scale, return on investment, health and welfare of the population, delivery of a healthy product, and so forth. Exotics veterinarians can leverage many of the same strategies used by their large animal veterinary counterparts to service their own patient population. Offering care on an ambulatory basis is among the most comprehensive ways to do so.[6] Benefits of ambulatory practice for reptiles and amphibians include the following:

Population health and welfare assessments

Like agricultural livestock, specimens in a herpetological collection can be examined as a "herd," an ambulatory visit essentially representing a nontraditional farm call. Animals in the collection are often kept in confined quarters and husbandry and infectious disease considerations relevant to one individual frequently apply to multiple animals within the group. Key cohorts, like quarantined animals, can be examined in situ without having to transport them off the premises.

Assessment of husbandry parameters and records

Husbandry practices play a crucial role in population health, especially for reptile and amphibian patients where most disease states have a basis in husbandry errors or stress. Rather than relying on the owner's report of husbandry conditions, ambulatory visits afford the practitioner the opportunity to observe husbandry conditions first-hand and allow a review of the client's recordkeeping. For example, temperature/humidity parameters can be collected and compared against the client's measurement equipment and perceptions. Enclosure cleanliness can be assessed and water from aquatic habitats can be collected for water quality testing on-site. UVB output can be directly measured from relevant lighting fixtures and recommendations given regarding distance of bulbs to bask sites. Location of and adequacy of enclosures—size and shape, substrate, ventilation, hides, cage furniture, ventilation—also can be assessed (and even corrected) during the visit.

Limit transport stress on the patient or collection of patients

Reptiles and amphibians are notorious for hiding clinical signs until becoming critically ill, and of course it is typically at this point that they are presented for examination. Ambulatory visits may allow the clinician to identify errors in husbandry or signs of disease earlier, and thus to intervene before patients become clinical. Because husbandry-related problems and stress are significant contributing factors in captive reptile and amphibian disease states, ambulatory visits are also valuable because they minimize exposure to inappropriate temperatures during transport, as well as reduce the stress of removing the patient from its normal habitat.

Economic feasibility, veterinarian-patient-client relationship, and perception of value

At an ambulatory visit, clients can be charged hourly rather than by the number of animals seen. This ensures the practitioner is compensated fairly for his or her time while incentivizing the client to work efficiently and ensuring the client is not unfairly penalized for having a large collection of animals. The opportunity to work together collaboratively can help to create lasting relationships of tremendous value to both doctor and client. Just as in-house clients can become regulars, those served on an ambulatory basis may also become committed, long-term clients. This provides a tangible perception of value that can pay dividends in client trust, and is a more meaningful way of fulfilling the legal requirement of a veterinarian-client-patient relationship. Many herpetoculturists have traditional dog/cat pets that may represent future small animal clients for practices that see them, as most pet owners would prefer to take all their animals to the same veterinarian for care. For the brick-and-mortar practitioner providing service on an ambulatory basis, this is a great way to develop the doctor-client bond in a way that is personally meaningful and meaningful to the business.[7] Ambulatory visits also represent a value-added service for clients with disabilities, small children, or other needs that make traditional office visits impractical.

Pooled sample collection

An ambulatory visit allows the clinician to make an evidence-based decision about which samples from which animals are most relevant. In some cases, it may be reasonable to treat the population rather than individuals. Where clinically appropriate, some samples (eg, fecal) can be aggregated from multiple enclosures and examined together. This type of approach saves the veterinarian time, saves the client money, and helps ensure the collection is getting the appropriate medical attention it requires.

Evaluate exceptional patients and patient populations

Certain reptiles and amphibians cannot or should not be transported for evaluation and are far better suited for ambulatory care. Large bioactive terraria and paludaria, those that are heavily planted or contain elaborate water features, may prove challenging to move, and the move itself could be dangerous or disruptive to the habitat. Additionally, large tortoises or crocodilians, especially if kept in quantities, are more easily evaluated on-site than if they are moved en masse into a clinic. Venomous reptiles are one particular group that could represent a potential safety hazard or legal liability in a traditional brick-and-mortar setting, but can be evaluated on an ambulatory basis if the keeper and veterinarian are appropriately trained and prepared.

Disadvantages and Other Considerations of Ambulatory Practice

Although ambulatory practice affords many benefits to the veterinarian seeing reptilian and amphibian patients, it also presents a unique set of challenges. Some of these challenges are presented as follows, with commentary on how they can be overcome, or recast as opportunities.

Safety

Veterinary medicine is an inherently dangerous profession, but veterinarians take precautions every day to mitigate occupational hazards.[8] This is no different in an ambulatory setting, but there are additional considerations when working with reptiles and amphibians. Situational awareness is paramount, beginning with knowledge of the client, as well as the collection one will be visiting. The veterinarian should always operate with at least one technician or assistant; traveling alone is never recommended. In addition to reptile and amphibian pets, clients may have dogs or other free-roaming animals that could pose an ancillary safety risk. Ask the client to contain any pets that may represent a bite risk or distraction before arrival. Also verify whether any of the species you are expected to examine represent an increased occupational hazard. Venomous reptiles, large snakes, large monitor lizards, and crocodilians all represent potentially serious safety considerations. The clinician must be informed of these at the time the appointment is scheduled to prepare appropriately. The clinician is under no obligation to commit to an ambulatory visit that cannot be conducted safely, and has the right to cancel or leave at any time if the safety of the team is jeopardized during the visit. Asking appropriate questions before the visit, and arriving prepared on the scene, helps to ensure everyone's safety. It also allows the clinician to control the visit, instilling confidence and relief in the client who may be as anxious about the call as the veterinarian.

Preparedness

The ambulatory clinician can be as effective in the field as in the clinic. However, without the benefit of a hospital full of resources, careful planning and preparation are crucial to the success of a visit. For example, reptilian and amphibian venipuncture can be challenging, so thorough review of anatomy should occur before the appointment, especially if servicing unfamiliar species. The veterinarian also should ensure an adequate number of syringes, needles, culturettes and other supplies that might be relevant to the visit before arrival (**Box 1**). Most clinicians will not have access to a serviceable radiography unit of any value for small reptile patients, and not every practice has a mobile ultrasound (although they are invaluable if available). The clinician should be cognizant of any limitations and be transparent with clients about which services can be offered on an ambulatory basis.

Box 1

Services frequently offered by the ambulatory veterinarian. Many services can be offered on an ambulatory basis; however, there are some services that would be difficult or inappropriate to perform in the field and are better suited for referral or transportation to a standing facility

Services commonly performed on-site in an ambulatory setting

- Observation and assessment of the facility
- Observation of the basic husbandry setup of the patient
- Obtaining full history and information about the presenting signs
- Cageside physical examination and sample collection
- Sexing
- Venipuncture for blood analysis (eg, complete blood count, chemistry) at the laboratory or clinic
- Cytologic sample collection: impression smears, skin scrapings, fine needle aspirates (for field review with mobile microscope or evaluation at a lab or clinic)
- Treatment of ectoparasites (enclosures and/or individual animals)
- Assist or tube-feeding and demonstration
- Administration of fluids (by mouth, subcutaneous, intracoelomic)
- Sedation with injectable medications (see **Table 2**)
- Minor surgeries (eg, small biopsies, lancing abscesses, digit amputations, hemipenal impactions)
- Prescribing medications
- Writing interstate health certificates (in the United States)
- Euthanasia
- Gross necropsy and sample collection
- Recheck examinations and follow-ups from previous ambulatory or clinic visits

Services one should consider referring or transporting to a standing facility

- Any procedure requiring inhalation anesthesia
- Major surgical procedures (eg, coeliotomy, removal of cystic calculi, enterotomies, management of large abscesses or other masses, limb amputation, tail amputation on larger reptiles, surgical management of dystocia, ovariohysterectomy and neutering, plastronotomy, fracture repair)
- Radiographic evaluation
- Submitting laboratory samples for pathologic evaluation
- International health certificates

Setting appropriate expectations for clients is paramount. It may also be difficult to anticipate and carry medications for dispensing. Transport of controlled drugs represents a legal "gray area," of which the ambulatory clinician should be aware. Clinicians should ensure that their liability insurance will cover potential loss or damage during patient transport. Although ambulatory care does come with some limitations, the veterinarian should not view these as failures, but rather as opportunities to recommend further evaluation in the hospital or offer referrals to better-equipped colleagues. The ambulatory practitioner also can offer to transport the patient on the client's behalf, providing a value-added service to the home visit.

Scheduling

Scheduling poses a challenge to ambulatory practitioners. Because there are more variables outside the veterinarian's control, site visits can run longer than antici- pated. If the appointment schedule is full when one visit runs late, it can create a domino effect in which the clinician runs late to every subsequent appointment. There are a variety of ways to schedule successfully that venture into the realm of practice management, which is beyond the scope of discussion here, but the au- thors have found some general guidelines helpful in reptile and amphibian ambula- tory practice.

○ Consideration should be given both to the type of animals to be examined, as well as the reason(s) for the visit. A client reporting mites, an outbreak of severe respiratory disease, or other potentially transmissible pathogen should not be scheduled before an afternoon of wellness visits. Similarly, the client who also runs a rodent-breeding operation may not be the client best serviced immediately before examining a collection of inquisitive tree monitors.
○ Any visits that will require extra care and attention to details (eg, venomous species) should always be scheduled with buffer time built-in. These appoint- ments should never feel rushed, as carelessness could have serious consequences.

As ambulatory visits become a regular part of practice, they run smoother and more efficiently. The short-term frustrations pay dividends as the practice grows.

Billing

These challenges are not unique to reptile and amphibian ambulatory practice, but providing estimates and setting clear expectations for payment before the appoint- ment can go a long way in ensuring a smooth visit. The authors recommend asking clients to pre-pay over the phone for the anticipated cost of their examination, which is billed hourly, in addition to a mileage fee. Logistically, clinicians typically limit calls to within a certain geographic area, and calculation of a mileage fee helps eliminate appointments accidentally booked outside a serviceable zone. Clients are made aware that the practice keeps track of visit time and bills accordingly. For appoint- ments completed faster than the time billed, credit can be applied toward diagnos- tics, retail, or other services provided at the visit or in the future. If the appointment runs late, clients can expect to be billed for the additional time with the cost of diag- nostics or other services rendered during the visit. Clients always receive a call from a client services representative the same day for collection of final payment by phone, and the total is never a surprise, as the ambulatory technician carries a lami- nated price list of regular diagnostics and services to keep the client updated during the visit.

Procedural compliance

There are unique legal and procedural considerations for the ambulatory practi- tioner who services reptiles and amphibians. For example, the possession and transport of these species are frequently regulated by local and regional govern- ments, so the veterinarian who services these patients should be familiar with all applicable laws. Additionally, veterinarians providing import/export services in the United States must be US Department of Agriculture–accredited Category II vet- erinarians through the National Veterinary Accreditation Program.[9] If the veteri- narian is providing an exclusively exotic house call practice, most states require

Table 1
Equipment of use to the ambulatory herptile veterinarian

Required	<ul><li>Disposable nitrile examination gloves</li><li>Unscented hand sanitizer</li><li>Gram scale patients and bathroom scale</li><li>Infrared/laser thermometer</li><li>UV meter</li><li>Sexing probes with water-based, nonspermicidal lubricant</li><li>Tape measure and/or calipers</li><li>Multiple bite blocks and specula of various sizes</li><li>Small vials of isopropyl alcohol and/or chlorhexidine scrub</li><li>4 × 4 gauze pads</li><li>Nail trimmers (small and large) and styptic powder</li><li>Syringes: 1.0, 3.0, and 6.0 mL</li><li>Syringe needles: 25, 22, 20, and 18 gauge</li><li>Portable sharps container and disposable trash bags for medical waste</li><li>Laboratory tubes for blood samples: heparinized with and without wax separators</li><li>Culturettes</li><li>Glass microscope slides, cover slips, slide carriers</li><li>Small vials, bottles, and syringes for dispensing medications</li><li>Prescription pad/booklet</li><li>Labels for medications (as required by state)</li><li>Pens/permanent markers</li><li>First-aid kit</li></ul>
Recommended	<ul><li>Doppler ultrasound with gel</li><li>Towels</li><li>Microscope</li><li>Camera</li><li>LED headlamp</li><li>Jeweler's loupes or other magnifying lenses</li><li>Instruments: small hemostats, suture removal scissors, forceps, needle drivers, sterile blade handles</li><li>Scalpel blades: No. 15 and No. 10</li><li>Sutures: 2-0 and 3-0 monofilament absorbable and nonabsorbable suture</li><li>Snake hooks and tongs</li><li>Examination gloves</li><li>Bottles of sterile saline</li><li>Bag valve mask with various endotracheal tube attachments for positive-pressure ventilation</li><li>Containers/bags for patient transport</li><li>Otoscope/ophthalmoscope</li><li>Ice chest for keeping medications/samples cool</li><li>Receipt booklet</li><li>Notebook</li><li>Business cards</li></ul>
Optional/ case-specific	<ul><li>Plastic tubes/shift box for venomous (or other) snake restraint</li><li>Welder's gloves</li><li>Face shield</li><li>Dremel tool and attachments</li><li>Syringes: 12 and 20 mL</li><li>Surgical pack and drape</li><li>Surgical gloves</li><li>Mobile ultrasound</li><li>Portable oxygen tanks</li></ul>

a written arrangement with a standing facility at which a practitioner may perform certain procedures, such as radiology, submission of laboratory samples, surgeries, and, possibly, drop-offs (including deceased patients) that cannot be offered on an ambulatory basis. Ambulatory clinicians servicing clients across state lines may need to be licensed by the state board in multiple states. Review of all applicable state practice acts and a consultation with a practice attorney is recommended.

Commonly Offered Services by the Ambulatory Herptile Veterinarian

The ambulatory practitioner is likely to encounter many of the same problems in the field that one would encounter in a hospital setting. Although some problems invariably require referral or transportation to a more appropriate or better-equipped facility, many traditional services can be offered, and many common problems addressed, on an ambulatory basis (**Table 1**).

Unless specified otherwise in one's jurisdictional practice act, there are no definitive rules governing what services can and cannot be offered on an ambulatory basis. Prudent clinical judgment is warranted and should be based on whether the procedure can be performed safely (to both patient and those present), expeditiously, and with access to follow-up in the event of complications.

Equipment and Supplies of Use to the Ambulatory Herptile Veterinarian

Each practitioner will have to determine what equipment and supplies are suitable and appropriate to take to an ambulatory call. Some items may be carried into the home or facility, whereas others can remain in the vehicle to be available on an as-needed basis. Medications and laboratory samples should never be left in a vehicle without providing refrigeration for storage.

The authors perform frequent ambulatory calls for herptile owners and have found a commercial fishing tackle box or portable toolbox (**Fig. 2**) useful for organizing an assortment of supplies. This equipment is summarized in **Tables 1** and **2**.

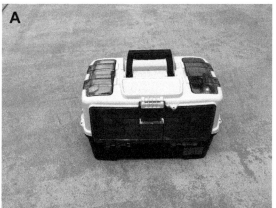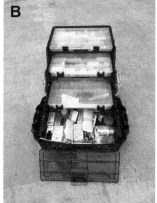

Fig. 2. A simple tackle box can be an effective way of transporting equipment for use at an ambulatory visit. (*A*) Small and portable when closed, most will (*B*) expand and offer immense organizational options built-in. (*Courtesy of* Richard Funk, MA, DVM, Mesa, AZ.)

Table 2	
Pharmaceutical considerations for the ambulatory herptile veterinarian	
Oral	• Meloxicam • Tramadol • Trimethoprim-sulfa (TMS) • Clindamycin • Enrofloxacin or orbifloxacin • Fenbendazole • Metronidazole
Injectable	• Ceftiofur • Ceftazidime • Danofloxacin • Alfaxalone • Dexmedetomidine • Atipamezole • Ketamine • Lidocaine/bupivacaine/mepivacaine • Meloxicam • Flunixin • Atropine • Epinephrine
Topical/- Environmental	• Neomycin/polymyxin/bacitracin ophthalmic ointment • Neomycin/polymyxin/dexamethasone ophthalmic ointment • Tobramycin ophthalmic drops • Oxytetracycline ophthalmic drops • Nystatin/neomycin/triamcinolone ± thiostrepton ointment • Silver sulfadiazine (SSD) cream • Manuka honey

SUMMARY

Herpetoculture continues to grow in popularity, a trend that has steadily gained momentum since the 1980s. Although the veterinary profession has evolved to keep pace with this growth, boasting many new advances in medicine and surgery, practice owners have been largely reluctant to break with norms based in small animal practice. These business practices are becoming less relevant and less appropriate for many modern reptile and amphibian collections. Practitioners willing to break with convention may find a more applicable model in production medicine, in which herptile livestock are evaluated on a population basis in an ambulatory setting.

Ambulatory medicine offers many advantages over outpatient care for veterinarians who see a reptilian and amphibian patient population. From the clinical benefits of evaluating patients and their living conditions in situ, to eliminating transport stress, to building client relationships, and tethering the growth of one's practice to that of an ever-growing industry, patients, clients, and practitioner alike all benefit in different ways from an ambulatory care option. Although there are some clinical problems better addressed in a controlled hospital setting, many common procedures in reptiles and amphibians can be performed in the field with readily available equipment that can be easily transported in a cooler, tackle box, and truck. Although ambulatory practice does come with some logistical challenges, most are overcome with time and experience, and these long-term benefits make the initial headaches worthwhile. Ambulatory practice represents a viable alternative to the traditional outpatient hospital visit model, one in which reptile and amphibian patients are particularly well-served.

REFERENCES

1. Mader DR, Mader-Weidner BS. Understanding the human-reptile relationship. In: Mader DR, editor. Reptile medicine and surgery. 2nd edition. St Louis (MO): Saunders Elsevier; 2006. p. 14–23.
2. Collis A, Fenili R. The modern U.S. reptile industry. Georgetown Economic Services, LLC; 2011. Available at. https://usark.org/wpcontent/uploads/2013/02/The_Modern_US_Reptile_Industry_05_12_2011Final.pdf. Accessed June 9, 2018.
3. Stoutenburgh GW. Building a successful reptile practice. In: Mader DR, editor. Reptile medicine and surgery. 2nd edition. St Louis (MO): Saunders Elsevier; 2006. p. 1–8.
4. Grand JA, Lloyd JW, Ilgen DR, et al. A measure of and predictors for veterinarian trust developed with veterinary students in a simulated companion animal practice. J Am Vet Med Assoc 2013;242:322–34.
5. AAHA-AVMA canine preventive healthcare guidelines. 2011. Available at: https://www.avma.org/KB/Resources/Documents/caninepreventiveguidelines_ppph.pdf. Accessed December 12, 2017.
6. AAHA-AVMA feline preventive healthcare guidelines. 2011. Available at: https://www.avma.org/KB/Resources/Documents/felinepreventiveguidelines_ppph.pdf. Accessed December 12, 2017.
7. Ramey DW. Equine ambulatory practice: challenges and opportunities. Vet Clin Equine 2012;28:1–9.
8. United States Department of Labor. Bureau of Labor Statistics 2010 Data. 2010. Available at: http://www.bls.gov/iif/oshwc/osh/os/ostb2801.pdf. Accessed February 26, 2018.
9. United States Department of Agriculture, Animal and Plant Health Inspection Service, National Veterinary Accreditation Program. 2018. Available at: https://www.aphis.usda.gov/aphis/ourfocus/animalhealth/nvap. Accessed February 26, 2018.

Avian Ambulatory Practice

Richard Gregory Burkett, DVM, DABVP (Avian Practice)

KEYWORDS

- Avian ambulatory practice • Mobile practice • Avian practice • Legal issues
- Business plan • Start-up costs • Marketing • Vehicles

KEY POINTS

- Avian veterinary medicine is a niche discipline that is an excellent choice for an ambulatory practice.
- Working with avian patients requires less space than with nonavian patients, an advantage when working inside a vehicle.
- Laws vary with each state and are regulated by that state's veterinary medical board.
- The importance of a business plan when starting an avian ambulatory practice is presented, including descriptions of the primary sections of a business plan.
- Information about vehicles available for avian ambulatory practices is presented, including descriptions of specific and customized features and the average cost of each vehicle.

INTRODUCTION

Ambulatory services have long been an important veterinary service provided to clients and their companion birds. Avian ambulatory services can be provided as part of a stationary avian practice or by an ambulatory-only avian practice. Avian ambulatory services are more often provided by an ambulatory-only practice. Starting an avian ambulatory practice is an easier and more affordable alternative to starting a stationary practice and, for this reason, is generally appealing to associates, relief veterinarians, and new graduates who want to open their own practice.

DEFINING AN AVIAN AMBULATORY PRACTICE

Avian specialty veterinary medicine is a niche discipline that lends itself as an excellent choice for an ambulatory veterinary practice. The foundation of an avian ambulatory practice is a vehicle that is designed, customized, and equipped specifically to fit the needs of an avian ambulatory practice. Avian ambulatory practice vehicles provide only a limited amount of space, which must be used efficiently to accommodate the

Disclosure: Owner and operator of The Bird Hospital: Avian Veterinary Services, The Birdie Boutique, Inc, Durham, NC.
The Bird Hospital: Avian Veterinary Services, The Birdie Boutique, Inc, 3039 University Drive, Durham, NC 27707, USA
E-mail address: drb@thebirdvet.com

equipment, supplies, and workspace needed to operate an ambulatory avian practice. Avian patients are well suited for an ambulatory practice because they tend to be smaller than the vast majority of nonavian patients, requiring less space. Along the same lines, avian patients weigh less, which allows for the use of a tabletop scale instead of needing a large space-occupying floor scale.

Space requirements for an avian ambulatory practice are also lower because some of the services that are traditionally offered in nonavian practices are not offered in an avian ambulatory practice. For example, bathing services and, for obvious reasons, dental care are not provided, which eliminates the need for a large associated equipment. An ambulatory practice is an affordable, practical, and effective option for practicing avian specialty medicine. It is a viable option to provide full-service avian medicine that is affordable as a start-up practice, operates with lower expenses, and has the capabilities of generating an excellent income.

ADVANTAGES AND DISADVANTAGES OF OPERATING AN AVIAN AMBULATORY PRACTICE
Advantages of Operating an Avian Ambulatory Practice

Two major advantages of operating an avian ambulatory practice are lower overhead costs and lower operating expenses compared with a stationary avian practice. In general, overhead expenses are fixed costs and operating expenses are variable. The advantage of lower overhead and operating expenses produces a higher profit margin.

An ambulatory avian practice is typically a 1-doctor practice, which has the advantage of allowing practitioners the autonomy of operating a practice at their own discretion. Solo practitioners working for themselves in an ambulatory avian practice have the flexibility to set their own schedule, which gives them the freedom to attend conferences, plan time for vacations and other recreational activities, spend time with their kids, or just take a day off.

There are advantages of an ambulatory avian practice for clients as well. The flexibility of a practitioner's schedule makes it easier and more convenient to schedule appointments. Clients generally prefer that their birds do not have to be placed in a carrier and transported to their veterinarian and reverse this process on the return trip; this is especially true for clients needing to transport multiple birds. An avian ambulatory practice is also convenient for those clients who are less mobile because of age or disability.

The advantage to the patients is that they tend to experience less stress when seen in the home environment where they feel secure. Clients are more relaxed when they see that their bird is less stressed and comfortable.

Avian ambulatory veterinarians can take advantage of home visits to view patients' environment and living conditions. Husbandry, basic care, cage set up, and cage placement within a client's home all have an effect on a bird's health. Adjusting these environmental factors can improve the bird's health and quality of life.

Disadvantages of Operating an Avian Ambulatory Practice

Solo practitioners in an avian ambulatory practice have only themselves to answer to, with the advantage of having freedom to decide what is best for their business and when they need to work. This situation also has its disadvantages. Solo practitioners are the only source of income for their practice, which can restrict the freedom to decide when they want to work. When solo practitioners are not working, there is no revenue generated. Time off comes at the expense of no pay.

Large stationary practices have the advantage of economy of scale. The disadvantage to small practices like an avian ambulatory practice is that they are not able to purchase supplies in quantities that allow for these discounted rates. A potential solution is for practitioners to work with their base hospital and place orders with them to enjoy their discounted rates.

Solo practitioners in an ambulatory avian practice must keep overhead costs low and frequently do so by limiting the number of employees on the payroll. These practices often have no employees. With fewer employees, practitioners must rely on themselves to perform the duties that otherwise would be the responsibility of employees. Practitioners become responsible for booking appointments and other receptionist duties; financial management, such as accounting, billing, and collections; and inventory management. These responsibilities add pressure to the job and take time away from practicing, which can lead to dissatisfaction with their career, and burnout.

An alternative to operating a practice without support staff is to employ a full-time technician who can reduce the practitioner's workload, thereby reducing the stress and pressures experienced when the practitioner bears all the responsibilities of practice management. A full-time technician in an ambulatory avian practice can provide the relief practitioners need to allow them time to focus on practicing medicine, managing patients, and writing records. One disadvantage to employing a full-time technician is increased overhead costs. Practitioners have some level of obligation and responsibility for ensuring that a full-time technician has the opportunities to work and earn a living. This is likely to impose restrictions to the scheduling freedoms enjoyed by self-reliant solo practitioners. Employing a full-time technician relinquishes some the practitioner's duties and responsibilities but adds the duty of employee management to the practitioner's list of responsibilities. Responsibilities associated with employee management include hiring and firing, payroll management, and scheduling. It is the decision of the practitioner to determine if the advantages of employing a full-time technician make up for the disadvantages associated with having a full-time technician.

Practitioners in an avian ambulatory practice travel the majority of the day, driving from appointment to appointment and potentially experiencing traffic delays. Contending with traffic can be a disadvantage when operating an avian ambulatory practice. Strategic route planning and appointment scheduling can prevent or reduce time spent sitting in traffic. For example, route planning that avoids major highways and avoiding scheduling appointments during peak driving times are necessary but require forethought.

Avian ambulatory practices often see patients in surroundings familiar to the bird, which is an advantage to the bird. This can be a disadvantage, however, for the practitioner. In familiar environments, especially in the presence of the owners, birds are more difficult to handle; they often become defensive and maybe even aggressive. These issues can be avoided if an avian ambulatory practice has a walk-in vehicle where the bird can be examined in an unfamiliar environment, without the owner present, if necessary.

THE LEGALITIES OF OWNING AND OPERATING AN AVIAN AMBULATORY PRACTICE

When starting an avian ambulatory practice, it is important to comply with state laws regarding owning and operating an ambulatory veterinary practice. The laws governing ambulatory practices vary by state. The North Carolina Veterinary Practice Act requires that ambulatory, mobile, and house-call practices that do not provide full-service veterinary care inform clients in writing which services are not available. North Carolina law also requires that if ambulatory practices do not provide hospitalization, emergency services, or radiology services, there must be a written agreement with a local clinic or hospital for the provision of these services. The name and address of the local clinic or hospital that is providing these services must be posted in plain view. The Act also states that ambulatory practices are subject to the same minimum standards as stationary practices.[1]

Licensed veterinarians are required by law to have a Drug Enforcement Agency license to administer and dispense controlled substances. The Controlled Substances Act prohibits ambulatory practices from transporting, administering, and dispensing controlled substances beyond their registered clinic locations. On July 16, 2014, the Senate approved an amendment to the Controlled Substances Act, the Veterinary Medicine Mobility Act (HR1528) that authorized ambulatory practitioners to carry controlled drugs away from their registered locations.[2]

THE IMPORTANCE OF A BUSINESS PLAN WHEN STARTING AN AVIAN AMBULATORY PRACTICE

A successful business begins with a good business plan. As with any new business, starting an avian ambulatory practice should begin with a thorough well-conceived business plan. The process of writing a business plan helps determine the feasibility of starting and maintaining an avian ambulatory practice. If it is determined that the practice could be successful, the next step is to procure funding. Typically, funding is through a bank loan, and some banks require a business plan as part of a loan application. The major sections that make up a business plan are the executive summary, industry analysis, company summary, marketing plan, and financial plan.

Business Plan: Executive Summary

The business plan should begin with the executive summary, which includes a mission statement and a list of goals necessary to achieve before starting a successful avian ambulatory practice. It also describes the business concept and an overview of the business model and explains why the business is uniquely qualified to succeed.

Business Plan: Industry Analysis

The industry analysis is a description of the state of the industry and industry trends. An industry analysis provides a market overview, an estimation of the market size, an analysis of the competition, and a description of the demand for the business.

Business Plan: Company Summary

The company summary provides a detailed description of the business and includes a description of the vehicle, licensing requirements, organizational structure, qualifications of the employees, and the management strategy of the practice. The company summary also provides inventory sourcing and description of the products and services and describes the needs of the clients.

Business Plan: Marketing Strategy

An avian ambulatory practice must be marketed properly to be successful. The marketing plan is vital to the business plan and to the success of the practice. It should be written as a plan for starting an avian ambulatory practice and as a long-term planning strategy to grow the practice and maintain and improve client retention.

Business Plan: Financial Projections

The financial section of the business plan is a complete and detailed account of the financial information pertinent to starting and operating an avian ambulatory practice. It is the primary section of the business plan that helps to determine the feasibility of starting and maintaining an avian ambulatory practice. It highlights the capital investment required to open an avian ambulatory practice and provides a list of funding sources that are available to the practitioner. The financial plan also projects operating expenses and gross revenue.

VEHICLE OPTIONS FOR AN AVIAN AMBULATORY PRACTICE

There are several types of vehicles that can be used for an avian ambulatory practice. The options are box inserts; chassis-mounted units; pull-behind bumper-hitch trailers and gooseneck trailers; box trucks; and recreational vehicles (RV). Although box inserts and chassis-mounted units can be used for an avian ambulatory practice, adapting and using them for this purpose is awkward, inconvenient, and inefficient. These types of units are typically designed specifically for large animals and farm calls.

Resourceful veterinarians also have the option of repurposing a used vehicle like a food truck. A food truck is an excellent vehicle to convert into an avian ambulatory vehicle because it already has plumbing and electricity, a refrigerator, and a freezer and may have stainless steel countertops.

Box Inserts

A box insert is used to convert a regular vehicle into one that is suitable for a mobile veterinary practice. The average cost for a box insert is $3000.[3] Box inserts are made to fit SUVs, pickup trucks, crew cab trucks, and vans. They are designed to carry only the essential equipment and supplies, which limits avian services that could be offered. Box inserts are available in several styles and offer a variety of well-organized shelves, compartments, cubbies, and drawers for easy access to supplies. Most models come standard with a water tank and pump, electrical outlets, and interior and exterior lighting, and the box insert is climate controlled. Large units provide similar standard features but have more storage and workspace.

Chassis-Mounted Units

Chassis-mounted units provide even more space and come with additional features, including refrigerators, hot and cold water, and large locking compartments to accommodate valuable equipment, such as a portable radiograph or ultrasound unit. The average cost for a chassis-mounted unit is $20,000.[3]

Pull-Behind Trailers and Motorized Walk-in Units

Pull-behind trailers are walk-in units that are towed and can not move on their own power. Box trucks and RV-type vehicles are walk-in units that are motorized and driven under their own power. These types of vehicles cost on average from $100,000 to $250,000.[4] The primary difference among different walk-in type vehicles is size. Pull-behind trailers are generally approximately 5m to 7m long, whereas the RV-type units can be up to 40 ft long. Standard on nearly all the walk-in types of vehicles are hot and cold water, electric generators, cabinetry and countertop space, examination table, hospital cages, 110-V outlets, and fresh water and gray water storage. The larger units come fully self-contained with all the features of a stationary veterinary practice. They have central vacuums; central heating, ventilation, and air conditioning

(HVAC) climate control; large refrigerator and freezer; full surgical suite with surgery lights and anesthesia machine; autoclave; digital radiograph unit; and laboratory equipment, including a blood analyzer, microscope, and centrifuge.

The walk-in types of vehicles are spacious and better suited for an avian ambulatory practice. They provide the opportunity to see avian patients inside the vehicle instead of inside a client's home. Being able to work inside the vehicle the veterinarian has all the necessary equipment and supplies conveniently available within a workspace that is designed specifically for avian patients. Avian patients tend to be less self-confident and easier to handle when they are in the vehicle outside their comfort zone.

Interior Design Considerations for Walk-in–Type Avian Ambulatory Practice Vehicles

Walk-in–type avian ambulatory vehicles provide the advantage of being able to see patients inside a vehicle. A major disadvantage is the risk of a patient escaping while being transported from the home to the vehicle. When handling an avian patient inside a vehicle, precautions should be taken to prevent accidentally releasing the avian patient, allowing it to be loose inside the vehicle. The disadvantage is if loose in the vehicle, an avian patient can retreat underneath a cabinet, on top of a cabinet, or behind an appliance, making retrieval of the patient difficult. There is also the risk of the patient escaping to the outside through an open door when loose inside a vehicle.

A vehicle that is customized for an avian specialty ambulatory practice should have features that reduce the risk of a patient escaping to the outside and make it easier to retrieve a patient that is loose inside a vehicle. One design feature is to ensure that all openings underneath and above cabinets and behind appliances and the entrance into the vehicle cab are blocked. This feature prevents patients from retreating to places that are difficult for the veterinarian to access. A second design feature is a safety area, which is an enclosed area that prevents the door in the vehicle from being open to the outside when entering and exiting the vehicle. The safety area is installed inside the vehicle around the exit door and can be made simply of a frame covered with screen or netting with a slit opening held closed with magnets or other type of closure. The enclosed area between the 2 doorways, the exit door of the vehicle, and the opening into the safety area need to be large enough for someone to turn around in and accommodate a patient's carrier. The safety area is entered through one doorway, which is closed once inside the safety area. The second door can then be opened without the danger of a patient escaping to the outside through the open exit door of the vehicle. A third feature is a barrier, like an accordion-style folding wall, that encloses the examination area when it is being used, thereby both reducing the risk of escaping through an open door and confining a loose bird to a smaller area.

As the fourth feature, the examination area should have bright lights that are controlled by separate controls that turn lights off and on independent from other lights in the vehicle. Lighting in the examination area needs to be very bright for a practitioner to better examine patients and to allow patients the ability to see well in the examination area. A separate light control allows practitioners turn lights on and off independently of other lights in the vehicle. The ability to turn lights off in the examination area is beneficial when removing a difficult-to-catch bird from its carrier or retrieving a bird that is loose inside the vehicle. Birds have near-zero ability to see in dim lighting; with the lights off, a practitioner can approach a bird unseen and be able to capture a patient safely, quickly, and efficiently.

Avian patients are unique in many ways compared with all other types of patients. Most unique is the ability to fly. Even in a small examination room, birds can fly around, which makes patients difficult to capture. Capture becomes even more challenging when a bird can perch or hang onto something out of reach of the practitioner. Landing also provide the patient an opportunity to rest, which rejuvenates the ability to continue playing chase. A fifth feature should be to keep the walls bare of all wall hangings, such as picture frames, to prevent patients from landing out of reach and resting.

STARTING AND MANAGING AN AVIAN AMBULATORY PRACTICE

An avian ambulatory practice has low start-up costs and can be a profitable business when managed properly. Scheduling and route planning help maximize the number of clients an avian ambulatory practice can see in a day and help keep expenses low. Properly managing expenses and generating the maximum amount of income by seeing as many patients as time allows generates profits that sustain and grow the practice.

Start-up Costs

The cost of opening an ambulatory avian practice is far less than the cost of opening a stationary avian practice. A stationary practice can cost approximately $1,000,000 or more to open.[4] An ambulatory practice can cost approximately $250,000.[4] The costs can be higher or lower depending primarily on the cost of the vehicle and equipment. Start-up costs to open an avian ambulatory practice include the vehicle and associated costs, equipment, supplies, and the opening inventory for dispensing and retail sales. The major expenses are the vehicle, licensing and insurance on the vehicle, and signage decals on the vehicle.

Overhead Costs and Operating Expenses

Overhead and operating expenses for an avian ambulatory practice are important factors to consider when determining the feasibility and profitability of a practice. An ambulatory avian practice is not burdened with the higher overhead and expensive operating costs of a stationary avian practice. Primary overhead and operating expenses for an ambulatory avian practice include the vehicle payment, vehicle licenses and taxes, vehicle maintenance and repairs, fuel, base-hospital usage fees, and employee payroll. Employee costs are often small and many have no employees other than the veterinarian.

Vehicle payments, insurance, taxes, service, maintenance, repairs, and inspections are essential operating expenses. The vehicle is the most important piece of equipment used in an avian ambulatory practice, and it must be maintained properly to keep it operational and safe to drive. An ambulatory avian practice cannot operate without a vehicle, and downtime means no income.

Fuel is another major operating expense in an ambulatory avian practice. The expense generated from fuel usage varies based on the price of gasoline and the vehicle's gas mileage. The vehicle's gas mileage is an important consideration when choosing a vehicle for an ambulatory avian practice. Research needs to be done to determine, for example, if diesel fuel costs more or less than regular gasoline and calculating cost per mile. Operating expenses generated from fuel usage can be kept to a minimum by choosing a vehicle with low gas mileage, shopping for the lowest fuel prices, and planning routes to use fuel efficiently.

An ambulatory avian practice is required by law in some states to have a base hospital from which to operate. Most, if not all, base hospitals charge a flat fee for their facilities and additional fees to use equipment. This expense for an avian ambulatory practice is generally only a small percentage of total overhead costs.

Equipment, Supplies, and Pharmaceuticals

The size and type of vehicle dictate how much and which equipment can be accommodated. Walk-in vehicles are capable of accommodating more equipment than box inserts and chassis-mounted units. Smaller walk-in units may only be able to accommodate a blood analyzer, centrifuge, microscope, and laptop computer. Larger walk-in units can accommodate more equipment, including digital radiograph systems, ultrasound machines, endoscopic equipment, and autoclaves.

An avian ambulatory practice is a specialty practice that requires specific equipment to provide the specialized care avian patients need. The equipment a practitioner chooses to use in an avian ambulatory practice is dependent on the vehicle and the services a practitioner wants to provide. The equipment needed to provide full-service avian medicine is listed in **Table 1**. The list of required equipment, recommended equipment, and optional equipment changes based on the level and types of services being offered by the avian ambulatory practice.

Table 1
Equipment used in full-service avian ambulatory practices

Required	Recommended	Optional
Anesthesia equipment: induction masks, nonrebreathing circuit, oxygen tanks, vaporizer, oxygen flow meter, endotracheal tubes, waste gas scavenger system	Electrosurgery equipment	Blood lead analyzer
	Heated surgery table	CT scanner
	Intravenous fluid infusion pump	Platelet-rich plasma therapy equipment
Anesthesia patient monitoring equipment	Nebulizing hospital cages	Stem cell therapy equipment
Autoclave	Oxygen therapy cages	Ultrasonic instrument cleaner
Blood chemistry analyzer	Patient positioner	
Centrifuge	Ultrasound system	
Computer system with redundant backup capabilities	Ventilator	
Digital radiography equipment		
Endoscopic equipment		
Fluid warmer		
Gram scale, 1–2 g increments		
Heated hospital cages		
Label printer		
Magnifying loupes and light		
Microscope		
Necropsy instrument kit		
Ophthalmoscope/otoscope examination magnifiers and lights		
Oral speculum, variety of sizes		
Oxygen source (tank, concentrator, or generator)		
Record-keeping system		
Rotary grinding tool (Dremel)		
Stainless steel gavage feeding needles, variety of sizes		
Stethoscopes		
Suction machine		
Surgical equipment: instruments, sterilizing containers, instrument markers		

Supplies needed to operate an avian ambulatory practice are much the same as those needed for an avian stationary practice. General supplies are needed for daily operations and are usually independent of the services being offered. Avian-specific supplies are usually not manufactured and are unavailable, but general use supplies are often modified to accommodate avian-specific needs. A list of general supplies is found in **Table 2**.

Table 2	
Supplies used in full-service avian ambulatory practices	
General	**Additional Description and Information**
Autoclave sterilizing supplies	Sterilizing envelopes, indicator strips, indicator tape, pack wraps
Bandage materials	2 in size may need to be cut into a narrow strip for small avian patients
Blood collection tubes	Microtainer tubes, most type commonly used in avian ambulatory practices
Blood transfusion supplies	
Chlorhexidine and iodine surgical scrubs	
Cleaning and disinfecting supplies	Mild avian-safe chemicals
Cotton balls	
Cotton-tip applicators	
Fluid administration and extension sets	
Fluids (normal saline and lactated Ringer solution)	Small-volume bags are preferred, avian patients are treated with small amounts of fluids; large bags tend to wasted
Gauze	
Iodine and betadine solutions	
Isopropyl alcohol	
Intravenous and butterfly catheters, variety of sizes	25 G, 22 G; limited need for 20 G, 19 G, and 18 G are the most used in an avian ambulatory practice
Laboratory testing equipment supplies	
Needles	Gauges: 27 G, 26 G, 25 G, 22 G, and 20 G; limited need for 19 G and 18 G; smaller gauges preferred from avian patients
Pharmaceutical dispensing supplies	Pill bottles, liquid bottles, prescription labels, mortar and pestle, oral dosing syringes, Flavorx compounding syrups; small and medium containers and oral dosing syringes are most used in an avian ambulatory practice
Red rubber catheters	All sizes
Sharps containers and biohazard bags	
Styptic	$AgNO_3$ or styptic gel (powder styptics are less effective and messy
Surgery supplies	Suture material, sterile gloves, masks, caps, gowns, drapes
Syringes, variety of sizes	1 cc tuberculin, 1 cc, 3 cc, 6 cc, 10 cc, 20 cc, 35 cc, 60 cc
Towels, variety of sizes	The safest method of capture

In any practice, pharmaceuticals are vital for treatment and management of disease. There are a limited number of pharmaceuticals used in avian medicine. Pharmaceuticals used in avian medicine are the same drugs that are used in other species. There are no medications that are labeled specifically for use in companion avian patients. The economics of pharmaceuticals, however, is different in an avian practice compared with other types of practices. Avian patients tend to be much smaller than nearly all other types of patients. Therefore, the quantities of drugs dispensed and administered to avian patients are also less. Nearly all pharmaceuticals are distributed in larger quantities than can be used in avian patients before the expiration date. This problem leads to large amounts of drugs being unused and discarded. A list of the general categories of pharmaceuticals and corresponding specific drugs is in **Table 3**.

Employees

An avian ambulatory practice can operate with many fewer employees than a stationary practice. Typically there is not a need to for a practice manager, a receptionist, and other support staff, which dramatically reduces the cost of payroll, payroll taxes, and employee benefits. A solo veterinarian or a veterinarian with an assistant or technician is typically sufficient staff to operate an avian ambulatory practice.

Route Planning and Time Management

As a business, an avian ambulatory practice needs to make a profit to be sustainable. The amount of profit made depends on the cost of doing business and the amount of gross revenue that is generated. Time is the limiting factor for generating income in an

Table 3
Pharmaceuticals used in full-service avian ambulatory practices

General Pharmaceutical Category	Specific Drug
Antibiotics	Ampicillin, amoxicillin, amoxicillin/clavulanate, cephalosporins, clindamycin, doxycycline, enrofloxacin, gentamicin, marbofloxacin, metronidazole, piperacillin/tazobactam, spectinomycin, sulfamethoxazole/trimethoprim
Antifungal	Amphotericin B, enilconazole, fluconazole, itraconazole, nystatin, voriconazole
Analgesic	Buprenorphine, butorphanol, hydromorphone, lidocaine, tramadol
Anti-inflammatory	Meloxicam, carprofen, dexamethasone, robenacoxib
Anesthetics and sedatives	Sevoflurane, midazolam, diazepam
Parasitacides and protzoacides	Albendazole, fenbendazole, ivermectin, metronidazole, pyrantel pamoate, praziquantel, sulfadimethoxine
Antiseizure	Diazepam, midazolam, levetiracetam
Miscellaneous	Sucralfate, albuterol, acetylcysteine, atropine, epinephrine, furosemide, flumazenil, heparin, mannitol, lactulose, milk thistle, ophthalmic drops and ointments (antibiotics, anti-inflammatory, barium sulfate suspension, Metamucil, leuprolide acetate, deslorelin implants, hyaluronidase, avian polyomavirus vaccine
Antitoxins	Activated charcoal, calcium EDTA, dimercaptosuccinic acid (DMSA), atropine
Nutritional supplements	Calcium gluconate, vitamins A/D, vitamin B complex, vitamin C, vitamin E/selenium

avian ambulatory practice; only so many clients can be seen in a day. A solo practitioner in an avian ambulatory practice has the freedom to determine how many hours each day to work. The more hours worked, the more clients that can be seen, thereby generating more revenue. Extending clinic hours allows practitioners more time to maximize the number of appointments they can see in a day. The number of appointments can also be maximized while keeping expenses low by holding clinics at apartment complexes and in neighborhoods. Planning routes can also maximize the number of clients as well as reduce travel time, driving distance, and fuel consumption. Additionally, route planning helps practitioners stay on time and be prompt to appointments, which contributes to a good reputation.

Record Keeping

Space is an important consideration in an avian ambulatory practice, and it must be used efficiently when practicing from an ambulatory vehicle. Nor only are medical records necessary to practice good medicine but also law requires them and requires that records be kept for a certain period of time. Paper records accumulated over time, occupying valuable space in an ambulatory avian practice. Operating as a paperless practice using a laptop computer that can remotely connect to a home system or a base hospital saves valuable space. Outside laboratory results can be received by email, and hard copies can be scanned into the system and discarded. Today, everything can be digital, including consent forms and laboratory request forms. Often there is a need to print discharge instructions, care sheets, and other information for clients or copies of medicals records for hospitals that have not advanced into the digital age. In situations where distribution of hard copies is necessary, compact portable printers can be used.

MARKETING AN AVIAN AMBULATORY PRACTICE

Marketing is a term that refers to a multitude of ways to promote an avian ambulatory practice. A good marking strategy uses several different types of promotions that are aimed at a target audience, which for an avian ambulatory practice is bird owners. The goals of a marketing plan are to generate revenue from current clients and grow the practice by generating new clientele. An effective marketing plan is a critical part of operating a successful avian ambulatory practice.

Advertising

Advertising is only one type of marketing used to promote an avian ambulatory practice. Types of advertising include radio ads, television ads, billboards, and electronic and print ads. Types of print media include newspapers, magazines, telephone books, entertainment programs and playbills, restaurant menus and placemats, promotional flyers, business cards, and reminder cards. Specialized niche services like an avian ambulatory practice rarely benefit from advertising in newspapers and most other print media because these forms of advertising do not reach the intended target audience. Printed promotional materials like flyers and reminder cards, which are typically distributed through direct mail using the US postal service, effectively reach the intended target audience. A printed brochure that gives detailed information about the practice is a good way to introduce the practice. Use this marketing technique to inform clients and potential clients of the services offered by the ambulatory practice, provide a map of the area covered, list diagnostic capabilities, and note the base hospital that is used by the ambulatory avian practice. Printed ads in bird industry trade magazines and other bird industry–related publications can be effective because they also reach the intended target audience. Most bird industry publications, however, have a national distribution. As such, even though these ads reach an intended audience, they likely attract only a small number of local readers, which means the average cost per new client generated is higher than print ads in less widely distributed publications. Bird industry–targeted print advertising can be cost-effective depending on the style of ad published. Large, colorful, full-page ads are not cost-effective. Small business card–sized ads are inexpensive, however, and although they may still attract only low numbers readers, the cost is low enough that attracting only a few new clients makes this type of advertising cost-effective. Other types of advertising, such as radio ads, television ads, and billboards, do not reach the intended target audience and are typically cost prohibitive.

Word-of-Mouth Marketing

The power of word of mouth for promoting an avian ambulatory practice should not be underestimated. Practices exist that thrive and grow on word of mouth only, with no form of advertising except a practice Web site.

The bird community is small, and bird owners often know many other bird enthusiasts. Veterinarians can generate a significant amount of business with word-of-mouth promotion but do not have direct control of this form of promotion. Happy clients tell friends about their experience with the practice; unhappy clients tell many more bird owners about their experience.

Electronic Advertising Using Email and the Internet

Email communications and Internet advertising are more cost-effective forms of marketing than print media. Email communications can be sent to groups of clients, or personalized email messages can be sent to individual clients. Internet ads reach globally, but target audiences also can be reached by placing ads on bird industry–related Web sites. The Internet has become a powerful marketing tool. Even though it provides worldwide distribution of ads and information, local readers can use the Internet to search for local avian veterinary care like they once used the telephone book yellow pages. Today, the Internet has been developed the ability to target individual people and present to those individuals tailored advertising, showing specific products and services of direct interest to those readers. Internet ads are also excellent for promoting a hospital's Web site and retail ecommerce site.

The most remarkable and effective system for disseminating ads and information over the Internet is through social media, which is expansive communications between and among other readers through Web sites designed specifically for person-to-person and person-to-people communications. Social media has become a worldwide phenomenon and opens the door to the largest audience that a practitioner can present advertising to. Essentially social media is the most effective word-of-mouth advertising.

Email communications are essentially free other than time and can be used to send reminders, promotions, coupons, newsletters, and educational information. Email has several advantages over print media. Email messages reach the audience almost instantly, which enables a faster response from clients. Email is environmentally friendly, which is attractive to most clients and establishes good will for the practice. Email messages can be used to send personalized messages to clients, such as updates on their hospitalized bird, or inform them of laboratory results. This kind of service is attractive to clients and generates a strong veterinarian-client bond.

Internet advertising is used to effectively distribute low-cost promotions to large audiences. Because the Internet is engaging and interactive, it is a powerful marketing tool and is a vital part of a strategy for promoting a modern avian ambulatory practice. It can be used in several of ways. A good use of the Internet is to publish a Web site for the avian ambulatory practice. It can be used to provide information about the practice/practitioner and clients can interact by using the Web site to schedule appointments and access educational material. A Web site can also be used for a retail ecommerce site to sell bird products, which generates additional streams of income for the practice.

Another effective use of the Internet is to place ads for promoting the practice and the ecommerce site. Internet ads are easily edited and can be updated and changed immediately, making it an excellent media for advertising. Internet ads are inexpensive enough to put up several different ads on multiple Web sites and get the most from a marketing budget. There are many Web sites that cater specifically to bird groups, providing many opportunities to promote an avian ambulatory practice.

Visibility Grows a Practice

The success of an avian ambulatory practice depends on having a client base large enough to sustain the practice and acquiring enough new clients to grow the practice and offset attrition. Marketing is basically making a practice visible to as many potential clients as possible using all available and relative types of promotions.

The vehicle is an effective marketing tool: it can be a traveling billboard by adorning it with decals of bright colorful birds and practice contact information, including a telephone number, practice logo, and Web site address (**Fig. 1**). If done creatively, this marketing tool can generate a significant amount of new business for the practice. One creative design style is to place decals in a way that gives a 3-D effect, such as a bird hanging from a part on the vehicle. Another clever design is to place decals on windows so the birds appear to be passengers in the vehicle (**Fig. 2**). The goal is for the avian ambulatory practice vehicle to be remembered and be a reminder that avian ambulatory medicine is available and who provides these services. A clever slogan or motto can help to keep a practice in the minds of potential clients (**Fig. 3**). A vanity license plate is another marketing tool that can make it easier for potential clients to remember a vehicle; most everyone likes to figure out the meaning of the letters and numbers on vanity license plate (see **Fig. 3**).

The vehicle is the first thing that a client sees either on the road or when it arrives. For this reason, it is important to keep the vehicle clean. If it is dirty and unkempt on the outside, the assumption could be that it is a reflection of the inside.

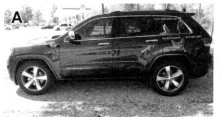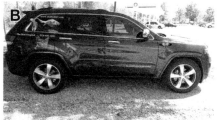

Fig. 1. Vehicles can be adorned. (*A*) Brightly colored decals that draw attention to your practice and market services. (*B*) The colorful decals are meant to highlight hospital name, phone number, and Web site address. (*Courtesy of* FCA US LLC, Auburn Hills, MI; and Greg Burkett, DVM, Durham, NC.)

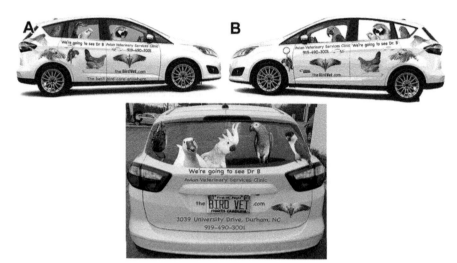

Fig. 2. Creative designs increase the effectiveness of this marketing strategy. (*A*) This vehicle takes advantage of a design with 3-D effects; for example, it is designed to have birds appear to be passengers, a passenger peering from behind another avian passenger, and the conure hanging from the fuel tank lid. (*B*) The birds in flight and the running chicken give the illusion of activity. (*C*) 3-D effects are attractive and draw attention, often as a double-take look. The cockatoo is behind the goose, the Congo gray is perched on the wiper, the caique is sitting on the edge, and the lory is hanging from the roof. 3-D effects on this vehicle promote a fun and happy practice by having the goose look like he is hanging out of the rear window with a smile. (*Courtesy of* Greg Burkett, DVM, Durham, NC.)

Visibility targets audiences and generates clients. Park, with permission, at a pet store or stationary nonavian veterinary hospital when it is necessary to stop and work on records or make client phone calls. Partner with these businesses to

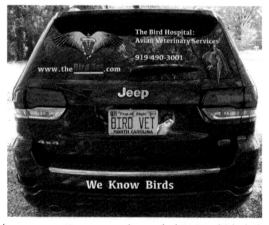

Fig. 3. A catchy slogan or motto on an avian ambulatory vehicle helps potential clients remember that these services are available and who provides them. "We know birds" and "the best bird care anywhere" are good slogans that can easily be remembered and associated with the avian ambulatory practice. Vanity plates are another effective strategy to help potential clients remember a vehicle, name, and services. (*Courtesy of* FCA US LLC, Auburn Hills, MI; and Greg Burkett, DVM, Durham, NC.)

exchange referrals and hand out business cards and practice brochures. An avian ambulatory practice can also partner with groomers, pet sitters, and dog walkers; practically any pet care business can be an excellent source of new clients.

SUMMARY

Some veterinarians have the hope of eventually owning their own practice. Opening a traditional veterinary practice requires a large investment, which may be unattainable. An ambulatory avian practice may be more appealing because it can be started with a substantially lower investment. Successfully opening an avian ambulatory practice begins with a sound business plan. Making an avian ambulatory practice successful requires a good marketing strategy. Practitioners need to use all the resources available. Standard marketing includes business cards, brochures, reminder cards, and trade magazine ads. Effective marketing is also accomplished with email communications and Internet ads. Another effective marketing tool is to adorn the vehicle with decals of colorful birds and the practice contact information. An avian ambulatory practice has advantages over a traditional practice. Seen by many as an advantage to operating an ambulatory avian practice, practitioners can be their own boss and set their own hours. Practitioners also enjoy the advantage of being able to work more intimately with their clients and patients. The primary disadvantages are that the solo practitioner has fewer employees to share duties with and they are the only source of income. If a practitioner does not work, then there is no income. This can contribute to being overworked and cause a practitioner to develop dissatisfaction with that career. Despite any of the disadvantages discussed, an avian ambulatory practice can be profitable and worth the investment.

REFERENCES

1. Veterinary Medical Board NC. The North Carolina Veterinary Practice Act, General Statutes of North Carolina, Rules and regulations, Article II, Chapter 90, Chapter 66, Section .0200, Rule. 0208 Facilities Providing Limited Veterinary Services, North Carolina Administrative Code. Available at: http://www.ncvmb.org/content/laws/documents/PRACTICE_ACT_PF.pdf. Accessed October 1, 2017.
2. Cohn T. Veterinary mobility act becomes Law. In: AVMA in the News. 2014. Available at: http://atwork.avma.org/2014/08/02/veterinary-mobility-act-becomes-law/. Accessed August 2, 2014.
3. Kelly C. Mobile vets are driven to succeed. In: Veterinary Practice News. 2011. Available at: https://veterinarypracticenews.com/mobile-vets-are-driven-to-succeed/. Accessed June 9, 2011.
4. Kramer MH. How to start a mobile veterinary clinic. In: Veterinary Practice News. 2017. Available at: https://www.thebalance.com/how-to-start-a-mobile-veterinary-clinic-125506. Accessed August 11, 2017.

Exotic Companion Mammal Ambulatory Practice, Including Potbellied Pigs and Llamas

Jane E. Meier, DVM

KEYWORDS

- Exotic companion animals • Potbellied pigs • Llamas • Ambulatory medicine
- Equipment • Restraint • Zoonoses

KEY POINTS

- Exotic companion mammal ambulatory practice has distinct advantages and disadvantages.
- Exotic companion mammal ambulatory practice is flexible with many ways to structure staff, territory, range, practice vehicle, support, scheduling, equipment, and services.
- Exotic ambulatory practice must comply with regulations relating to the mobile nature of the practice.
- Appointments, examinations, diagnostics, treatment, and euthanasia are uniquely challenging in an ambulatory exotic mammal practice.
- Zoonoses must be considered when working with nontraditional species of mammals.

INTRODUCTION

Ambulatory exotic companion mammal practice is a rewarding and challenging aspect of veterinary medicine. There are as many ways to organize a mobile practice as there are different veterinarians. Mobile practice is well suited to veterinarians who are calm, flexible, and enjoy improvising and developing novel ways of doing things. It is rarely boring, and no 2 days are alike.

ADVANTAGES

Car rides, changes in ambient temperature, nonroutine handling, and strange sights, sounds, and smells are all stressful to healthy exotic animals and more so to an ill individual. Prey species and wildlife are especially vulnerable to these disruptions, and

Disclosure Statement: The author has nothing to disclose.
3048 Bonita Mesa Road, Bonita, CA 91902, USA
E-mail address: JEMEIER@AOL.COM

Vet Clin Exot Anim 21 (2018) 651–667
https://doi.org/10.1016/j.cvex.2018.05.004

nondomestic animals hide weakness especially well when stressed. These traits, coupled with native behaviors, makes recognizing and identifying illness more difficult than diagnosing illness in domestic animals. Moving an ill or brittle exotic small mammal can make an animal's condition worse.

Husbandry and nutrition issues contribute to many medical problems. These issues are not readily discovered in an office setting. Because less is usually known about the husbandry and nutritional needs of exotic companion mammals than common domestic mammals, husbandry and nutritional problems are often more of an issue.[1] Because the veterinarian is dealing with only part of the puzzle (without firsthand knowledge of the animal's physical environment and daily routine), ambulatory services allow for empirical observations (**Fig. 1**).

Clients benefit from house calls if they do not have to take their animal(s) to the veterinarian.[2] Many potbellied pigs do not take kindly to car rides; chinchillas are sensitive to increased ambient temperatures where hot cars can cause thermal stress[2]; and whereas llamas normally take a trailer to transport, moving an entire habitat may be difficult if not impossible. If clients have multiple and/or large animals, do not drive, or are handicapped, transporting animals to a stationary veterinary clinic may be a hardship.

An onsite veterinary consultation provides better observations of husbandry, nutrition, temperature, habitat, sanitation, behavior, and group dynamics. A veterinarian can observe enclosures, cleaning, food preparation, and feeding. Over time, the emphasis can switch from treating individual problems to a proactive approach highlighting preventive medicine. Clients can learn from their veterinarian and vice versa with greatly improved abilities to provide medical care.

An ambulatory practice can be a nice addition to a stationary practice that already treats small exotic companion animals or wildlife. It can set the practice apart and offer another dimension of service. For a new practice, it is an easy way to get started, with lower overhead and startup costs as well as capturing a distinct, available market share. An ambulatory practice provides a more accurate and detailed view of the patient and its environment than what can be acquired in a standard brick-and-mortar practice setting.

The interpersonal relationship between clients and veterinarian is on a different footing with a mobile practice. Veterinary offices, like physician offices, can be intimidating and frightening to clients. Unlike a stationary practice, where the client is in the veterinarian's space and place of business, the veterinarian is in the client's space, which changes the dynamic. The veterinarian is a guest in the client's home or facility, and the cultural imperative of providing hospitality often comes into play. Clients are frequently more relaxed and understand and retain more of what a veterinarian tells them. The relationship between the veterinarian and client often evolves to more of a partnership or even friendship. Knowledgeable clients most commonly take pride in teaching veterinarians about their animals and the care that they provide.

DISADVANTAGES

Veterinarians in a typical small animal practice may spend 10 minutes to 15 minutes per patient for a routine examination. Most house-call appointments last at least 30 minutes. If assessment of management and husbandry is included, the call can take an hour or more. If a patient requires anesthesia, monitoring is required until it is sufficiently recovered to be safely left in the care of the owner. Travel time must also be factored into the duration of each call, resulting in fewer patients visited in a typical day than seen during the same time in a stationary practice. Fewer transactions means lower income for the veterinarian, but, critically, this can be offset by lower overhead.

To be economically sound, an ambulatory small exotic animal practice may need to charge as much or more than a stationary counterpart. Most clients using ambulatory services seem to think this is worthwhile for the individualized and comprehensive attention they receive.[1]

The limitations to what can be done in a home setting can be frustrating to both animal owner and veterinarian. Not having the luxury of a fully staffed and stocked hospital or the correct equipment, medication, or supplies can be a distinct disadvantage to a mobile practice. Space for equipment and supplies in a vehicle is generally limited. Forgetting an important item or not bringing duplicates of essential supplies can derail the call. A good ambulatory veterinarian quickly learns to build in redundancy and, with good planning and checklists, can easily learn to mitigate most, if not all, limitations.

Making a checklist of equipment and supplies of both items to take to an appointment and items to take away at the end of the call or having totes/carriers where common items have a designated location can reduce forgotten items.

STAFF

Some mobile practitioners work with no employees, preferring to do their own scheduling, ordering, cleaning, record keeping, restocking, driving, and so forth. Some use part-time veterinary technicians or other staff. Others have full-time technicians and support staff. Staff need to have many of the same characteristics that make a good mobile exotic mammal veterinarian. They need to be well versed in a variety of species and restraint techniques and be able to interact well with clients and patients. They need excellent technical skills and must be able to improvise. If they make appointments, they need to ask the right questions so appropriate equipment, supplies, and adequate time are allotted for patients. Extra staff may be employed when a complex or difficult procedure is planned.

SCOPE

A mobile exotic companion mammal practice can be an independent, stand-alone full-service practice. It can be an extension of the services offered by a stationary practice, or it can offer some services with referrals to full-service hospitals for procedures requiring anesthesia, imaging, critical care, or continuous monitoring. Many full-service stationary hospitals are open to referrals, partnerships, or affiliations because they view ambulatory exotic companion practice as an addition to their practice rather than competition. The practices are complementary.

When setting up a mobile practice, "What to do where?" is a critical question. The answer determines how the practice is structured. Will the services offered be restricted and limited to examinations and simple procedures? Will the practice offer onsite anesthesia, surgery, or imaging? Will patients be transported back to an existing stationary practice or referred to another practice?

Some companion mammal ambulatory practices are stand-alone practices with a self-sufficient full-service mobile clinic. Several manufacturers make full-service mobile veterinary clinics and trailers. (Two sources of veterinary clinics are La Boit Specialty Vehicles at http://www.laboit.com and Magnum Mobile Specialty Vehicles at http://magnummobilesv.com.). A standard class A or class B motorhome can be customized to the exact specifications of a practice. Businesses that do van conversions are likely take on the challenge of building an exotic companion animal clinic. Visiting recreational vehicle (RV) shows as well as veterinary conferences help acquaint veterinarians with the systems and options available in RVs. Purchasing an unfinished model allows for initial customization without having to remove the standard RV interior.

Slide-in, chassis-mounted, and insert mobile veterinary clinics are other options, especially if a practice has a limited scope (One source of mobile veterinary clinic inserts is Bowie at http://bowieintl.com.). The least expensive option is a practice vehicle with removable storage for veterinary supplies. Self-stacking storage bins are inexpensive and come in multiple sizes, can be partitioned, and are durable (One source of bin systems is American Van at https://www.americanvan.com/shelf-and-bin-systems/bin-system/self-stacking-bulk-storage-bins-example.html.). Although acquiring the supplies and equipment takes time, storage bins can easily turn a car into a mobile practice vehicle.

Some mobile practices advertise on their vehicles whereas others do not. It is an individual choice, with pros and cons. Advertising on the vehicle can increase business, but it can also invite break-ins by those looking for money, drugs, and veterinary equipment. Good security systems and safe overnight parking are considerations for any ambulatory practitioner.

TERRITORY AND RANGE

House-call veterinarians need to decide how far they are willing to travel to see clients. Time spent in transit is time lost seeing patients. Urban and suburban practices may not need to travel as far as rural practices.

FEE STRUCTURES AND STRATEGIES

Fee structures may be similar to those charged by a stationary exotic small animal practice for examinations, procedures, laboratory results, consultations, and so forth, with an additional call fee added. The call fee may be based on distance traveled from the home base or the transit time. Some veterinarians charge a premium for house calls. The call fee may be included with the examination fee or broken out separately. When working with large numbers of animals, charging by the hour plus costs may be more practical.

Do not make assumptions about what clients will spend to care for their exotic small companion animals. The value to a client may have no relationship to the monetary value or replaceability of the animal. Offer nonjudgmental options.

Acceptable payment methods should be determined and the mechanics of the payments put in place. Decide whether to accept cash, checks, credit cards, insurance, or charges on account in advance. Determine the mechanics of payment and where to safely store cash, if taken in the field. If credit cards will be accepted in the field, consider credit card readers that work with mobile phones. These units work on both Android and iOS phones and are small and convenient. (An example of card readers is Square at https://squareup.com/reader.). Some thought should be given to how and where to safely store cash, if taken in the field.

RECORDS AND REFERENCES

Some veterinary practice management software is specifically set up for ambulatory practice. A comparison of programs is an essential part of choosing practice management software.[3] Research the choices, talk to colleagues, test the software, ask questions, check the companies, and decide what features are important. Cloud-based or Internet-based programs may not be practical if the Internet or cellular service is inconsistent in the practice's geographic range. Some areas have reliable service and others do not.

Even with reliable service, computers, servers, hard drives, and batteries can fail. If practice management software is used, a backup paper system should be available for medical records, forms, releases, essential references and formularies, and pricing information. Canceling appointments because practice software or hardware is down is upsetting to clients and is not productive.

INSURANCE

Make sure the practice vehicle has adequate insurance. This should include liability, physical damage, collision damage costs, medical payments, and damage from a covered natural disaster. If the vehicle is used to transport patients, animal bailee insurance is recommended. The American Veterinary Medical Association/Professional Liability Insurance Trust recommends this optional endorsement if animals are hospitalized, boarded, or transported. It covers damage to animals resulting from fire, wind, theft, escape, flood, vandalism, attack from other animals, and many other perils not related to treatment (http://www.avmaplit.com/products/animal-bailee/).

REGULATORY
Veterinary Practice Act

Several state veterinary practice acts set minimum standards for mobile veterinary clinics and ambulatory practices. These standards are often revised and updated annually. Make sure the ambulatory vehicle is in compliance with the state veterinary practice and has the required permits. The minimum standards may be similar to the requirements for stationary practices. Other discussions on this topic are found in the Adolf K. Maas' article, "Ambulatory Exotic Animal Medicine Legal Issues," in this issue.

Medical Oxygen

Medical oxygen, or oxygen USP (United States Pharmacopeia) is considered both a hazardous material by the US Department of Transportation (DOT) and a prescription drug regulated by the US Food and Drug Administration. The law the DOT follows comes from title 49 of the Code of Federal Regulations sections 40, 382, 383, 387, 390 to 397, and 399.[4]

Transporting oxygen cylinders is regulated by the DOT and the Occupational Safety and Health Administration (OSHA). An oxygen manifest is normally required for transporting oxygen cylinders. The only exception to the shipping paper requirement is when the hazardous material is used as a material of trade. For example, welders, plumbers, or veterinarians are transporting the gas to a job site, where they will use the gas in the course of their work. That is considered a material of trade. Persons who fall under a material of trade exception are not selling their hazardous materials; they are selling their services.[5]

OSHA regulations in regard to transporting oxygen cylinders are as follows:

- 1926.350(a) (4)
  - When cylinders are transported by powered vehicles, they shall be secured in a vertical position.
- 1926.350(a) (5)
  - Valve protection caps shall not be used for lifting cylinders from one vertical position to another. Bars shall not be used under valves or valve protection caps to pry cylinders loose when frozen. Warm, not boiling, water shall be used to thaw cylinders loose.
- 1926.350(a) (6)
  - Unless cylinders are firmly secured on a special carrier intended for this purpose, regulators shall be removed and valve protection caps put in place before cylinders are moved.

- 1926.350(a) (7)
  - A suitable cylinder truck, chain, or other steadying device shall be used to keep cylinders from being knocked over while in use.
- 1926.350(a) (8)

  When work is finished, when cylinders are empty, or when cylinders are moved at any time, the cylinder valve shall be closed.[6]

Regulated Medical Waste

A mobile veterinary practice needs to comply with regulations for medical waste generators. Because rules vary by location, a copy of the medical waste regulations from appropriate jurisdictions should be obtained and reviewed to be certain of the correct disposal rules.

Ambulatory veterinary practices may need to get an exemption from regulations governing medical waste haulers. Transporting used syringes and needles, tissue, sharps, infectious animal waste, cultures, and other biohazard waste may require a permit to haul medical waste. Generally, the regulations about medical waste are written with stationary waste generators in mind (hospitals, veterinary practices, dental offices, laboratories, funeral homes, and so forth). Permitted third-party haulers move waste from the generators to disposal facilities. Make sure these regulations do not apply to an ambulatory practice. Check with state, county, or local waste regulators for guidance.

Controlled Substances

According to the Drug Enforcement Administration, practitioners are required to store controlled pharmaceuticals in a securely locked, substantially constructed cabinet.[7] Compact safes firmly bolted or welded to the vehicle work to secure controlled substances in a mobile setting. Placing the safe where it cannot be seen makes it more discrete and secure, but regulations are in flux and vary between the schedule of drug being carried. Further information regarding controlled drugs can be found in the Adolf K. Maas' article, "Ambulatory Exotic Animal Medicine Legal Issues," in this issue, and at the Drug Enforcement Administration Web site.

APPOINTMENTS
Preappointment Client Instructions

Instruct the client not to clean the patient's habitat the day before the appointment. Urine, feces, food, and bedding should be left in place and the patient should not be bathed. The client should be ready to demonstrate how and what the animal is fed. Always instruct the client to have the animal contained if they are free ranging because an animal that cannot be captured easily can destroy a busy work schedule. Some animals can be confined in a bathroom or other small room.

A pet carrier can be used for restraining and containing potbellied pigs. If a potbellied pig is not critically ill, have the owner feed only one-half the normal ration the day before the appointment. Food can be a strong motivator for pig compliance and cooperation, but use caution if anesthesia is planned during the visit.

Scheduling

Scheduling appointments for an ambulatory small exotic animal practice requires more preparation than scheduling for a stationary practice. The scheduler should try to group routine appointments in the same geographic area to save travel time. Estimating adequate travel time should allow for traffic, distance, roads conditions, weather, and time of day. Accurate address and directions are vital. With GPS applications, an accurate address and directions are less important; however, not all online

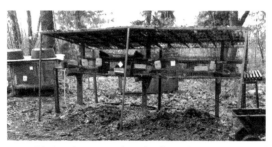

Fig. 1. A small home rabbitry that was described in the paperwork from the owner as "Excellent ventilation, with excellent protection from the weather, cleaned often with active social interaction between rabbits." This exemplifies the value of empirical observation. (*Courtesy of* Adolf K. Maas, DVM, Bothell, WA.)

maps are correct. Find out from the client if there are any tricks or tips to finding their location.

When deciding on the length of time to allot for the appointment and equipment or supplies needed, the scheduler should consider the following questions:

- What is the animal species?
- Are there any aggression issues with the animal?
- Is the animal able to be handled?
- What is the reason for the call?
- What is the history of the issue?
- Does the patient have multiple caretakers?
- Will it involve an in-depth evaluation of husbandry, behavior, or diet?
- Is this a first time visit or a recheck?
- Will vaccinations or injections be given?
- If so, will there be 10 minutes to 15 minutes postinjection to observe the animal for allergic or anaphylactic reactions?
- Will there be multiple animals to examine?
- Will the animal require sedation or anesthesia?
- If so, what will be the recovery time requiring veterinary monitoring?

The scheduler should be attuned to any strange or false signals from clients, especially clients unknown to the practice. Safety for the veterinarian and staff is of paramount importance. The veterinarian is going to a client's location that may be isolated and less controlled than a stationary practice. Unfortunately, drug seekers may target veterinarians and mentally unstable people can also be animal owners. As a precaution, a trusted person should know the veterinarian's daily call schedule. This is especially important if the veterinarian is a solo practitioner who works alone. Most cell phones have tracking systems that can relay a real-time location to a third party, and there also are apps that immediately contact emergency services on demand.

EQUIPMENT
Capture and Restraint

For handling most species, a gentle calm approach works best. Use the minimum restraint necessary to do the job safely for the people and the patient. Have clients condition their pets to being handled and restrained. Use positive reinforcement and short lessons. The owner can make a game of it. Food rewards can be great motivators, especially with potbellied pigs. Pigs have long memories and may be better at training their owners than vice versa.

Just as a puppy, kitten, or foal is taught to tolerate grooming and touch to the entire body, exotic small animals, potbellied pigs, and llamas can be conditioned to tolerate similar restraint and touch. Llamas can be aggressive if they have been hand raised or have too much human attention as crias.[8]

Animals can be trained to allow preventive procedures without significant restraint but work and planning are required by owners well in advance. In cases of a medical emergency or natural disaster, all animals need to have their own transport cage or carrier and be comfortable in it. Acclimation should be taught to animals by their owner/handler. Llamas, for example, need to readily load into a transport vehicle. If the client owns or can borrow a trailer, put it in the llama's pen and feed llama in it until it goes in and out easily.[3] The same can be done with transport cages or carriers used with any animal. The carrier should be a place of safety and refuge.

Small Companion Exotic Mammals

An exotic mammal practice requires some specialized capture and restraint equipment (**Fig. 2**). Sometimes chemical restraint or anesthesia is less stressful and easer for all involved than manual restraint.

When manual restraint is used, equipment may include any of the following:

- Assorted gloves—golf, work, animal handling, and cut proof
- Assorted sizes of cat restraint bags
- Ferret muzzle
- Assorted sizes of towels, blankets, and pillow cases
- Assorted nets, including fish and bird nets
- Leashes, ropes, and harnesses
- Squeeze or transfer cages (Two sources of cages are Livetrap http://livetrap. com/ and Wildlife Control Supplies https://www.wildlifecontrolsupplies.com)
- Tarps (visual barriers)
- Blowpipe or blowgun
- Catch pole
- Clear plastic restraint tubes—tube rodent holders (One source of restraint tubes is Kent Scientific at https://www.kentscientific.com.)
- Plexiglass anesthetic chamber
- Size-appropriate anesthetic face masks
- Size-appropriate endotracheal tubes
- Size-appropriate laryngoscope
- Portable inhalation anesthetic machine

Potbellied Pigs

Potbellied pig restraint equipment includes the following:

- Pig sorting panels or push boards (One source of push boards or sorting panels is Nasco at https://www.enasco.com.)
- Bucket—pigs can be backed into a corner with a bucket over their head
- Harness and lead—caution, some pigs can slip a harness
- Restraint chute (One source for restraint chutes is Shaul's Mfg at http://www. shaulsmfg.com.)
- Polyvinyl chloride (PVC) restraint chute—homemade with 4-in to 5-in PVC pipe and crosspieces to snuggly fit the pig. (It assembles like tinker toys. The bottom is open, and the chute is placed over the pig.)
- Sling—homemade from a tarp with leg cut out for each leg. Two, 5 cm by 10 cm wooden studs of approximately 2 meters in length (or equivalent) are attached to

the tarp edges so the supports run parallel to the sides of the pig. Walk the pig over the tarp, align the leg holes, and have several people lift the pig.
- Ear plugs for the handlers
- Size-appropriate face masks
- Large animal face mask - homemade from a 3.8 L bleach bottle
- Size-appropriate endotracheal tubes
- Laryngoscope with long blade
- Shopping cart restraint—useful for examinations of pigs up to 54 kg. Cover the top to prevent escape.[9]
- Forking - grooming and stimulating the pig with a fork along the back and flanks. Many pigs will lie down and allow examination, treatments, and hoof trimming as long as the stimulation continues.[10]

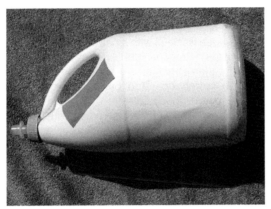

Fig. 2. A large bleach bottle can be modified into an anesthetic face mask suitable for pot-bellied pigs, large carnivores, and pinnipeds. A hole is drilled in the bottle cap, and an endotracheal tube connector is glued in place. The bottom of the bottle is cut out. The rim is covered with silicone tubing, which has been cut lengthwise and glued in place.

Llamas

Llama restraint equipment includes the following:

- Llama halter
- Ropes
- Crossties
- Blindfold or calming mask
- Commercial llama chute (One source for llama chutes is Light Livestock Equipment at https://www.lightlivestockequipment.com/product-category/chutes/.)
- Homemade llama chute (Two sources for plans for homemade llama chutes are Southwest Llama Rescue at http://www.southwestllamarescue.org/chute.html and Llama Life at http://llamalife.com/wp-content/uploads/2015/10/chuteplans.pdf.)

EXAMINATION AND DIAGNOSTICS

Space is limited in an ambulatory exotic companion mammal practice. Some specialized equipment is essential and should be included with the standard equipment for an exotic companion animal veterinary practice. A 12-V centrifuge, which can be run from the vehicle, allows blood and laboratory samples to be spun as soon as possible to avoid hemolysis or altered results from sitting or shaking in the vehicle. Micro–blood tubes are designed for small specimens. A portable glucose meter helps diagnose hypoglycemia or hyperglycemia on site. An ice chest or a 12-V cooler/heater can be used to keep specimens and medications cool or to warm fluids.

A portable, battery-operated gram scale (A source for a battery operated gram scale is SR Instruments at https://srinstruments.com/category/vet-avian-scales and a larger battery operated scale at https://srinstruments.com/category/vet-mobile-veterinary-scales.) are essential for monitoring patients and calculating appropriate doses. The weight of a potbellied pig can be estimated with a measuring tape.

Estimated potbellied pig weight (pounds)[11,12] = (length × girth × girth)/400 (inches)
    Length—measure from the base of the ear to the base of the tail (in inches)
    Girth—measure around the pig's body just caudal to the front legs (in inches)

Rechargeable or battery-operated clippers work even if there are no electric outlets handy. A pediatric stethoscope is useful with small animals. A light meter or light meter app for a mobile phone helps determine light levels, and laser-guided digital infrared thermometers or high-low thermometers are useful for determining environmental temperatures. Disposable battery-operated quick cautery units and silver nitrate sticks are an inexpensive means of hemostasis.

A hands-free headlamp, medical magnifier, and a powerful flashlight are necessities. Most household lighting is not sufficient for excellent visualization of small patients or those in poorly lit surroundings. A digital camera or phone application can be used to document medical problems, set baselines, and judge progress. An otoscope can be used for oral examinations, and specialized dental instruments are available for rodents and rabbits. An assortment of nail clippers, both human and animal, is useful for foot care. The nails of some animals can be trimmed through screen or cage wire. Potbellied pigs require farrier tools for hoof care. A battery-powered rotary tool is multipurpose and can be used on hooves, nails, and even teeth, with care and experience.

THERAPY

Always carry emergency drugs for treating anaphylaxis, shock, and cardiovascular emergencies. Keep dosage information simple and available. Anaphylaxis does not happen often, but when it does, be prepared. Make sure to give injections and vaccinations early in the visit so the patient can be observed for at least 15 minutes to 20 minutes for adverse reactions. Ferrets may be more prone to vaccine reactions than many other species. Do not leave the site until enough time has passed to preclude a severe reaction.

Killed or recombinant vaccines are safer for exotic mammals than modified live vaccines. Modified live vaccines have been attenuated and tested in the domestic species for which the vaccine was developed and these vaccines have not been tested in other species. As a concern, some modified live vaccines produce overt disease in other species. For example, one modified live canine distemper vaccine produced canine distemper in raccoons in a wildlife rehabilitation setting (Nikos Gurfield, DVM, DACVP, personal communication, 2011).

Build in redundancy and have duplicate supplies of critical items. Murphy's law applies to veterinary practice. The only bottle of inhalation anesthetic, tranquilizer, euthanasia solution, or antibiotic is the one that drops and breaks. The only sterile pack gets contaminated. The valve on the oxygen cylinder leaks. If it is critical to the job, it is well worth it to have a backup.

A makeshift incubator for neonates or critically ill animals can be made using an ice chest, a microwaved sock filled with dry rice or beans, and a digital thermometer to monitor the temperature. Be careful to keep the temperature in a safe range. Hypothermia or hyperthermia can result from inattention to the ambient temperature. If the animal is able to move, allow it to move to or away from a heat source. Put a heating pad under half the container or cage. Shine the heat lamp in a corner so the animal can choose its location.

Some 3/10-mL and 1/2-mL insulin syringes with 27-gauge or 28-gauge 1/2-in needles are excellent for injections in small patients. In addition, the needle can be pulled off with forceps or pliers, and the syringes can be used to accurately dose small volumes of oral medications (BD [Becton, Dickinson and Company, NJ, USA] Micro-Fine intravenous needle Units-100 insulin syringe, 1/2-mL or 3/10-mL, with 28-gauge × 1/2-in needle). A permanent marker or tape can mark syringes so clients know how much medication to administer. Do not assume clients know how to measure 1 mL versus 0.1 mL versus 0.01 mL.

Medication administration can be a challenge. Working with a good compounding pharmacy is helpful. It can compound most medications into flavors preferred by an animal and keep volumes low. If a patient cannot be handled easily, be creative. Oral medications can be hidden in favorite foods or treats or mixed into something sticky and placed on an animal's fur to be groomed off. When possible, pick medications that are given only once or twice daily. Less often is better.

WHEN TO STOP HANDLING

Veterinarians are taught to do no harm. When working with exotic small companion animals and wildlife, the veterinarian must remember that any handling can be stressful to these patients. Unlike domestic animals that may find comfort and enjoyment in close proximity to people, this is not the case with all exotic small companion mammals. Wildlife, in particular, find handling and proximity a threat and may respond as if it were a dangerous event.

Be aware of an animal's response to handling. Monitor fight-or-flight responses. There are times when it is better to put the animal away and come back to finish an examination, treatment, or procedure another time.[13] Keep handling sessions brief and monitor closely. Speak softly and preplan the procedure to keep handling time to a minimum. Covering a patient's eyes may be calming but do not become so focused on the task that the animal as a whole is forgotten. Sometimes sedation or anesthesia is safer even with the inherent risks because the stress response is dramatically attenuated, decreasing the overall risk to the animal.

EUTHANASIA

Euthanasia in a mobile setting requires skill, tact, and sensitivity. Clearly discuss the steps that will occur in detail and what the owner should expect. For instance, the animal's eyes may stay open and the animal may urinate or defecate. Reassure the owner that the animal's veterinarian is the animal's advocate and will make sure the animal is truly euthanized before the call is over and that the animal will not wake up later. Give owners the option to watch the euthanasia or leave the area, providing a supportive environment so they do not feel judged for whatever their decision is. It is recommended to tranquilize or anesthetize the animal prior to the euthanasia, smoothing the procedure for the pet, the owner, and even the veterinarian. Use humane procedures to perform the euthanasia, which can be found within the *AVMA Guidelines for the Euthanasia of Animals: 2013 Edition*.[33]

Table 1
Zoonoses in exotic companion animals, including potbellied pigs and llamas

Chinchillas	Dermatophytosis
	Lymphocytic choriomeningitis virus
	Baylisascaris procyonis
	Listeriosis
Chipmunks	*Yersinia pestis* (plague)
Ferrets	Salmonellosis
	Yersinia pestis (plague)
	Leptospirosis
	Dermatophytosis
	Influenza A and B
	Ectoparasites
	Cryptosporidiosis
	Giardiasis
	Campylobacteriosis
	Rabies
	Listeriosis
	Tuberculosis
Gerbils	Leptospirosis
	Ectoparasites
Guinea pigs	Balantidiasis
	Chlamydiosis
	Dermatophytosis
	Ectoparasites
	Lymphocytic choriomeningitis virus
	Salmonellosis
	Yersinia pseudotuberculosis
Hamsters	Salmonellosis
	Campylobacteriosis
	Dermatophytosis
	Ectoparasites
	Lymphocytic choriomeningitis virus
	Tularemia
	Leptospirosis
	Tapeworm
Hedgehogs	Salmonellosis
	Yersinia pestis (plague)
	Aphthae epizooticae (foot-and-mouth disease)
	Ectoparasites
	Cryptosporidiosis
Llamas	Rabies
	Parapox sp (contageous ecthyma)
	Dermatophytosis
	Tuberculosis
	Brucellosis
	Listeriosis
	Leptospirosis
Mice	Salmonellosis
	Yersinia pestis (plague)
	Rickettsia sp
	Hantavirus
	Lymphocytic choriomeningitis virus
	Dermatophytosis
	Ectoparasites
	Streptobacillus moniliformis (rat-bite fever)
	Leptospirosis

(continued on next page)

Table 1 (continued)	
Opossums (Virginia)	Leptospirosis
	Tularemia
	Erysipelothrix sp
	Trypanosoma cruzi (Chagas disease)
	Ectoparasites
	Dermatophytosis
	Tuberculosis
	Salmonellosis
	Rabies (rare)
Potbellied pigs	Rabies
	Tuberculosis
	Ectoparasites
	Balantidiasis
	Giardiasis
	Erysipelothrix sp
	Influenza
	Erysipelothrix sp
	Streptococcus group D
	Ascaris suum
	Leptospirosis
	Brucellosis
Prairie dogs	*Yersinia pestis* (plague)
	Monkey pox
Rabbits	Tularemia
	Enterohemorrhagic *E coli*
	Cryptosporidiosis
	Encephalitozoon cuniculi
	Pasturella sp
	Coxiella burnetii (Q fever)
	Dermatophytosis
	Ectoparasites
	Salmonellosis
	Tapeworm
	Campylobacteriosis
Rats	Salmonellosis
	Yersinia pestis (plague)
	Streptobacillus sp
	Rickettsia sp
	Hantavirus
	Ectoparasites
	Leptospirosis
	Lymphocytic choriomeningitis virus
	Streptobacillus moniliformis (rat-bite fever)
Skunks	Listeriosis
	Rabies
	Tularemia
	Leptospirosis
	Baylisascaris procyonis
	Baylisascaris columnaris
Sugar Gliders	Salmonellosis
	Giardiasis

Data from Refs.[14–32]

Mask the exotic small companion animal with inhalation anesthetic or use premedication sedatives, such as alfaxalone, butorphanol tartrate, and midazolam hydrochloride, in combination, subcutaneously or intramuscularly. These work especially well in virtually all small mammals. Intranasal midazolam followed by inhalation anesthesia, preceding intravenous or intracardiac injection of euthanasia solution, is an effective protocol in potbellied pigs.

The clinician needs to determine in advance if their practice provides body removal services, and, if so, which species/sizes will be attended. If these services are offered, be certain to carry appropriate bags or containers, securely label the body, and have a dedicated freezer of appropriate size to store remains. If this service is not offered, tell owners their options at the time the appointment is scheduled. If the euthanasia is elected during the appointment, discuss body care options prior to the euthanasia and have a list of service providers in their area. If a body pickup service is used, schedule it to come at least an hour after the scheduled veterinary appointment to decrease stress and emotions for the owner and to make sure the procedure is completed prior to their arrival. Some clients prefer to have the veterinarian make the arrangements, and others prefer to make their own plans.

The client and veterinarian may prefer handling the financial transaction prior to the euthanasia, rather than at the end of the call, as is typical for routine appointments.

ZOONOTIC POTENTIAL

Many zoonoses are described in exotic companion animal species (**Table 1**). For some of these zoonoses, there is proof of transmission to humans. In other cases, the potential for transmission is real. The same pathogen can induce clinical signs in humans and in animals. Zoonoses should be recognized and understood so the risks of transmission can be minimized. Mobile veterinarians are ideally placed to educate clients about zoonoses because they see the animal's environment, sanitation, and husbandry (**Fig. 3**).

Common sense and good hygiene and sanitation can mitigate much of the risk. Instruct owners to keep the animal and the environment clean. Everyone should wash hands with a disinfectant soap before and after handling animals. Animal handlers should avoid touching their face or mouth and change clothes if they become soiled. Wash animal bedding and food and water containers separately and use bleach or other strong disinfectant, if possible. Use disposable paper towels, not dish cloths, to dry hands, surfaces, and containers. Dispose of animal waste in a sanitary way. Immediately wash off saliva, blood, urine, and feces with a good disinfectant

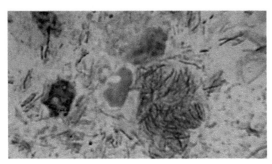

Fig. 3. Mycobacteria initially identified from a rat's skin lesion (acid-fast staining, ×1000 magnification.). (*Courtesy of* Adolf K. Maas, DVM, Bothell, WA.)

soap. Veterinarians have a responsibility to educate their clients about the dangers of zoonotic diseases and how to minimize those risks.

In addition to zoonotics, the ambulatory practitioner needs to be concerned about spreading disease from one stop to the next. Just as in dairy or swine medicine, the veterinarian has to be careful not to act as a fomite for disease, particularly when considering some species commonly carry bacteria that can cause serious to fatal disease in other species. Reverse zoonoses can also occur, such as human influenza infecting ferrets, so any time there is a health concern that is dealt with, whether prior patients or veterinarians themselves, appropriate sanitation, protection, and procedures need to be followed to prevent transmission.

ACKNOWLEDGMENTS

The author wishes to acknowledge the contributions of Alice J. Vranes, DVM; Regina M. Taylor, RVT; and Leslie Van Epps for their contributions to this article.

REFERENCES

1. Fisher PG. Equipping the exotic mammal practice. Vet Clin North Am Exot Anim Pract 2005;8:405–26.
2. Driggers T. The mobile exotic animal pet practice. Vet Clin North Am Exot Anim Pract 2005;8:463–7.
3. Howard B. Head-to-head battle of the PIMS. In: Veterinary economics. 2016. Available at: http://www.veterinarybusiness.dvm360.com/head-head-battle-pims. Accessed May 31, 2018.
4. 49 CFR parts 300-399. In: Federal Motor Carrier Safety Administration, United Stated Department of Transportation. Available at: https://www.fmcsa.dot.gov/regulations/title49/b/5/3. Accessed March 31, 2018.
5. Marquard V. DOT regulations for transporting oxygen cylinders. In: HomeCare Magazine. 2014. Available at: https://www.homecaremag.com/law/jan-2014/protect-your-company-following-dots-oxygen-provider-regulations. Accessed March 31, 2018.
6. Regulations (standards - 29 CFR) ßafety and Health Regulations for Construction. In: Occupational Safety and Health Administration. Available at: https://www.osha.gov/pls/oshaweb/owadisp.show_document?p_table=STANDARDS&p_id=10696. Accessed March 31, 2018.
7. Summary of Controlled Substances Act Requirements Appendix C. In: Practitioner's manual an informational outline of the controlled substances act, United States Department of Justice Drug Enforcement Administration Office of Diversion Control 2006. Available at: https://www.deadiversion.usdoj.gov/pubs/manuals/pract/appendices/app_c.htm. Accessed April 1, 2018.
8. Bennett M, Richards N. Camelid wellness. Vet Clin North Am Exot Anim Pract 2015;18:255–80.
9. George L, et al. Restraint of pigs. In: The new pot bellied pig manual 2012. Available at: https://www.vin.com/members/cms/project/defaultadv1.aspx?pId=5260&catId=6528&id=5260795&ind=17&objTypeID=17. Accessed March 30, 2018.
10. Sawyer B, Cox N. Forking fantastic welcome to forking 101. In: Mini Pig Info 2015. Available at: https://www.minipiginfo.com/forking-mini-pigs.html. Accessed March 31, 2018.
11. Davenport S. Mini pigweight loss plan - Welcome to fat camp. In: American Mini Pig Association. Available at: http://americanminipigassociation.com/

mini-pig-health/mini-pig-weight-loss-welcome-fat-camp/. Accessed March 31, 2018.

12. How to calculate pig weight using a measuring tape. In: Adapted from Washington State University. Available at: http://extension.oregonstate.edu/coos/sites/default/files/howtocalculatepigwtusingmeasuringtape.pdf. Accessed March 31, 2018.

13. Doneley R. Ten things I wish I'd learned at University. Vet Clin North Am Exot Anim Pract 2005;8:393–404.

14. Johnson-Delaney C. Safety issues in the exotic pet practice. Vet Clin North Am Exot Anim Pract 2005;8:515–24.

15. Pignon C, Mayer J. Zoonoses of ferrets, hedgehogs, and sugar gliders. Vet Clin North Am Exot Anim Pract 2011;14:533–49.

16. Hill W, Brown J. Zoonoses of rabbits and rodents. Vet Clin North Am Exot Anim Pract 2011;14:519–31.

17. Brust D. Sugar glider (petaurus breviceps) pet care. In: A quick reference guide to unique pet species 2011. Available at: https://www.vin.com/members/cms/project/defaultadv1.aspx?pId=12071. Accessed March 30, 2018.

18. Johnson-Delaney C. Virginia opossums pet care. In: A quick reference guide to unique pet species 2011. Available at: https://www.vin.com/members/cms/project/defaultadv1.aspx?pId=12071&catId=49805&id=6904838. Accessed March 30, 2018.

19. Bradley T. Pet rabbit care. In: A quick reference guide to unique pet species 2011. Available at: https://www.vin.com/members/cms/project/defaultadv1.aspx?pId=12071&catId=42776&id=6846200&ind=8&objTypeID=10. Accessed March 30, 2018.

20. Kiefer K, Johnson D. Pet ferret care. In: A quick reference guide to unique pet species 2011. Available at: https://www.vin.com/members/cms/project/defaultadv1.aspx?pId=12071&catId=42776&id=6853686&ind=9&objTypeID=10. Accessed March 30, 2018.

21. Johnson-Delaney C. Guinea pigs or cavie (cavia porcellus) pet care. In: A quick reference guide to unique pet species 2011. Available at: https://www.vin.com/members/cms/project/defaultadv1.aspx?pId=12071&catId=42776&id=6862768&ind=10&objTypeID=10. Accessed March 30, 2018.

22. Leck S. Hamster pet care. In: A quick reference guide to unique pet species 2011. Available at: https://www.vin.com/members/cms/project/defaultadv1.aspx?pId=12071&catId=42776&id=6864062&ind=11&objTypeID=10. Accessed March 30, 2018.

23. Leck S. Rat pet care. In: A quick reference guide to unique pet species 2011. Available at: https://www.vin.com/members/cms/project/defaultadv1.aspx?pId=12071&catId=42776&id=6865514&ind=12&objTypeID=10. Accessed March 30, 2018.

24. Leck S. Domestic mice (Mus musculus) pet care. In: A quick reference guide to unique pet species 2011. Available at: https://www.vin.com/members/cms/project/defaultadv1.aspx?pId=12071&catId=42776&id=6864848&ind=13&objTypeID=10. Accessed March 30, 2018.

25. Leck S, Johnson-Delaney C. Gerbil pet care. In: A quick reference guide to unique pet species 2011. Available at: https://www.vin.com/members/cms/project/defaultadv1.aspx?pId=12071&catId=42776&id=6867238&ind=15&objTypeID=10. Accessed March 30, 2018.

26. Leck S. Chinchilla pet care. In: A quick reference guide to unique pet species 2011. Available at: https://www.vin.com/members/cms/project/defaultadv1.

aspx?pId=12071&catId=42776&id=6873214&ind=16&objTypeID=10.   Accessed March 30, 2018.
27. Johnson-Delaney C. Hedgehogs (Atelerix albiventris/Erinaceus europaeus) pet care. In: A quick reference guide to unique pet species 2011. Available at: https://www.vin.com/members/cms/project/defaultadv1.aspx?pId=12071& catId=42776&id=6869543&ind=17&objTypeID=10. Accessed March 30, 2018.
28. Kramer M, Lennox A. Skunk pet care. In: A quick reference guide to unique pet species 2011. Available at: https://www.vin.com/members/cms/project/defaultadv1. aspx?pId=12071&catId=42776&id=6874453&ind=19&objTypeID=10. Accessed March 30, 2018.
29. Tynes V. Miniature (Potbellied) pig (Sus scrofa domestica) pet care. In: A quick reference guide to unique pet species 2011. Available at: https://www.vin. com/members/cms/project/defaultadv1.aspx?pId=12071&catId=42776&id= 6872313&ind=28&objTypeID=10. Accessed March 30, 2018.
30. Johnson S. Llama (Lama glama) pet care. In: A quick reference guide to unique pet species 2011. Available at: https://www.vin.com/members/cms/project/defaultadv1. aspx?pId=12071&catId=42776&id=6899894&ind=26&objTypeID=10. Accessed March 31, 2018.
31. Sinclair K. Richardson's ground squirrel (Spermophilus richardsonii) pet care. In: A quick reference guide to unique pet species 2011. Available at: https://www. vin.com/members/cms/project/defaultadv1.aspx?pId=12071&catId=42776&id= 6909528&ind=40&objTypeID=10. Accessed March 31, 2018.
32. Sinclair K. Flying squirrel (Glaucomys spp.) pet care. In: A quick reference guide to unique pet species 2011. Available at: https://www.vin.com/members/cms/ project/defaultadv1.aspx?pId=12071&catId=42776&id=6924738&ind=42& objTypeID=10. Accessed March 31, 2018.
33. AVMA Guidelines for Euthanasia of Animals. 2013 Edition. Available at: https:// www.avma.org/KB/Policies/Documents/euthanasia.pdf. Accessed May 31, 2018.

United States Department of Agriculture Facility Inspection for Exotic Veterinarians

Susan Horton, DVM

KEYWORDS

- USDA • APHIS • AWA • Accredited • Accreditation • Facility inspection
- Attending veterinarian • Program of veterinary care

KEY POINTS

- The attending veterinarian must be accredited.
- The attending veterinarian must have a formal arrangement with the facility.
- The Program of Veterinary Care is created by the attending veterinarian.
- Research facilities will require participation in the Institutional Care and Use Committee.

INTRODUCTION

Under the Animal Welfare Act (AWA), facilities that are licensed by the US Department of Agriculture (USDA)/Animal and Plant Health Inspection Service (APHIS) must have a relationship established with a veterinarian.[1] This relationship may be as a full, part, or contract Attending Veterinarian (AV). The AV should be familiar with the AWA, which was passed by Congress in 1966 and has been amended several times to include pertinent aspects.[2,3] It is currently under amendment at the time of this publishing. This act was developed to set general standards for humane care and treatment that must be provided for certain warm-blooded animals.[2] It is necessary that the veterinarian be accredited by the USDA/APHIS to provide signatory for the APHIS Form 7002.[2] Last, the veterinarian must be familiar with the necessary paperwork required by the USDA/APHIS.[1] Because this is for the situations addressing nontraditional species, cat and dog requirements are not discussed.

Disclosure: The author has nothing to disclose.
Chicago Exotics Animal Hospital, 3757 West Dempster Street, Skokie, IL 60076, USA
E-mail address: Chicagoexoticspc@gmail.com

Vet Clin Exot Anim 21 (2018) 669–684
https://doi.org/10.1016/j.cvex.2018.05.012
1094-9194/18/© 2018 Elsevier Inc. All rights reserved.

vetexotic.theclinics.com

WHY BE AN ATTENDING VETERINARIAN FOR A UNITED STATES DEPARTMENT OF AGRICULTURE LICENSEE OR REGULATED FACILITY?

The opportunity to be a full- or part-time AV for one of these situations brings interesting locations and situations. In other words, it brings you outside of the regular veterinary practice and presents new opportunity and experience. Part-time AVs can work this easily into their existing practice to increase revenue and bring in new clients. You may find yourself able to provide and ensure proper veterinary care to large numbers of unusual animals that would not necessarily be received in your existing practice. The education and experience needed as well as gained from these situations will benefit you and the animals that you examine and treat.

ACCREDITATION

The National Veterinary Accreditation Program (NVAP), established by APHIS in 1992, is managed nationally, but authorization is still managed on a state-by-state basis. This program has allowed for more organized administration of the program by standardizing the accreditation procedures and requirements.[4]

Veterinarians who wish to become accredited through this program must be a graduate with a Doctorate of Veterinary Medicine or an equivalent degree (any degree that qualifies the holder to be licensed by a state to practice veterinary medicine) from a college of veterinary medicine and also be a veterinarian that is licensed or legally able to practice veterinary medicine in the state in which the veterinarian wishes to perform accredited duties.[5] Next, they must take the Initial Accreditation Training (IAT). Each state will offer an Orientation Program following the IAT. There are 2 categories established for accreditation (category I and category II). Category I includes all animals except food and fiber species, horses, birds, farm-raised aquatic animals, all other livestock species, and zoo animals that can transmit exotic animal diseases to livestock. Category I animal species are limited to dogs, cats, laboratory animals (rat, mouse, gerbil, guinea pig, hamster), nonhuman primates, rabbits, ferrets, minks, gophers, amphibians/reptiles, and native nonruminant wildlife. Category II includes all animals. Examples are food and fiber animal species (cow, pig, sheep, goat, all ruminant), horses (mule, ass, pony, zebra), all bird species and poultry, farm-raised aquatic animal species, livestock species (bison, captive cervid, llama, alpaca, antelope, other hoofed animal), zoo animals that can transmit exotic animal diseases to livestock, as well as category I animals (eg, dogs, cats, small rodents). It is recommended that the AV be a category II accredited veterinarian.[6] Specific requirements exist for these categories, and they must be renewed every 3 years. In this way, specialization is provided for accreditation.[4] Accreditation is accomplished by completing educational units found at the veterinary accreditation Web site. Once the program is completed, the applicant must submit the application form VS Form 1-36A.[7] This form is submitted to the NVAP Coordinator. Once approved, the applicant will receive a certificate, an Accreditation Renewal Date, and a 6-digit National Accreditation Number.[4]

ROLE OF THE ATTENDING VETERINARIAN

The role of the AV is to uphold the standards of the AWA. Ensuring that the facility inspected is current within the regulations set forth by the AWA is a key factor. The AV will help the facility set up an adequate animal care program and should have expertise in the management of animals maintained in the facility. Supporting the animal care inspectors is also part of the AV's job.

The AWA has set guidelines for humane care and management of most warm-blooded animals. Included are warm-blooded animals bought and sold commercially as pets or for research. Animals that are exhibited to the public, such as zoos, circuses, educational demonstrations, and certain performances, are covered by the AWA as well, and these facilities must have appropriate certification. Also included are facilities in which animals are used in biomedical research, education, experimentation, or animals that are transported commercially.[2] Animals not covered by the AWA include farm animals raised for agricultural purposes, such as for meat, wool, milk. Horses and birds not used in research, mice (*Mus*) and rats (*Rattus*) used in research, fish, invertebrates, and cold-blooded animals (reptiles and amphibians) are not covered by the AWA.[1,2,8] Birds (other than those bred for research) are covered under the AWA, but the regulatory standards have not yet been established[8] (**Fig. 1**, **Table 1**).

A person who is a dealer, exhibitor, or breeder licensed under the AWA is called a licensee.[2] The facility where regulated animals are used in research or education, or someone who commercially transports animals, and experimentation is called a registrant.[2] The responsibility for complying with the AWA lies with the licensee and registrant.[2] The managing veterinarian associated with the licensee or the registrant is known as the AV.

A formal arrangement must be made between the licensee or registrant and the AV. In the case of a part-time AV, the formal arrangements must include a written plan on veterinary care and scheduled visits.[2] The animals will need daily assessment of their health and well-being. The AV will need a form of direct communication from the licensee or registrant on animal health, behavior, and well-being. The method of contact can be as easy as an e-mail and/or cell number where a member of your staff can communicate with the licensee. All communications need to be recorded in the permanent record, just as with any other medical case. E-mail exchanges are excellent because they are easy to add to the permanent record.

The AV should have expertise in the management, medicine, and care of the licensee or registrant's animals. Consultation with experienced veterinarians must be

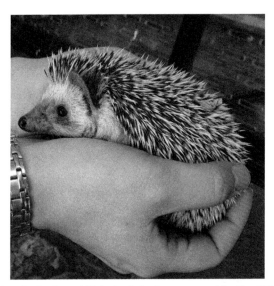

Fig. 1. North African hedgehogs (*Atelerix algirus*) are covered by the AWA.

Table 1		
Animals that are regulated by the Animal Welfare Act		
Not Covered by AWA	**Covered by AWA**	**Covered by AWA**
Birds not used in research	Alpacas	Coatis
Horses, donkeys, mules	Farm-type animals not used for	Kinkajous
Reptiles and amphibians	agricultural purposes	Wild/exotic canids
Farm-type animals used for	Foxes and mustelids	Megaherbivores (rhinos,
agricultural purposes	Wild or exotic hoofstock	Elephants, hippos,
Invertebrates	Opossums	giraffes)
Fish	Rabbits, raccoons, squirrels	Primates
	Zebras	Wallabies and kangaroos
	Camels	*Wild/exotic cats
	Common pet-type mammals	Bears
	Cavies	Pocket pets

Data from US Government Publishing Office. Animal Welfare Act TITLE 7 — AGRICULTURE Chapter 54; USCode 2013, 1290–1308. Available at: https://www.gpo.gov/fdsys/pkg/USCODE-2013-title7/pdf/USCODE-2013-title7-chap54.pdf.

arranged if the AV determines their experience is insufficient. Training and further education should be considered by the AV in such cases. Seeking qualified education through an RACE (Registry of Approved Continuing Education)[9] -approved program held in the area needing improvement or mentorship by a qualified veterinarian will help the AV offer more complete service. Occasionally a facility may use more than one AV[1] because the AVs may have different areas of expertise. Having multiple veterinarians involved underscores the need for accurate and complete record maintenance. Whether employed on a part-time or consulting basis, formal arrangements and specific areas of authority must be documented and agreed by all parties involved[1] (**Box 1**).

PROGRAM OF VETERINARY CARE AND ANIMAL AND PLANT HEALTH INSPECTION SERVICE FORM 7002

The program that the AV must create should include all health-related aspects of veterinary care. Detailed descriptions of managing animal health, monitoring and preventing disease, employee knowledge, and husbandry will need to be part of the written program. The plan should also include a plan for after hours, holiday, and

Box 1
Responsibilities of the attending veterinarian
• Establish and maintain the PVC
• Conduct regular visits to the premises, if the AV is part time or a consultant who is the AV
• Develop and maintain a written PVC, if the AV is part time or a consultant
• Provide guidance to personnel on all animal-related activities
• Establish and maintain the method or methods of euthanasia for the animals, which should be consistent with the current AVMA Guidelines on Euthanasia (https://www.avma.org/KB/Policies/Documents/euthanasia.pdf)

Data from United States Department of Agriculture (USDA). Animal Welfare Inspection Guide. USDA. 2013. Available at: https://www.aphis.usda.gov/animal_welfare/downloads/Animal-Care-Inspection-Guide.pdf. Accessed November 1, 2017.

weekend situations when medical care is needed. This comprehensive document is known as the Program of Veterinary Care (PVC). A portion of the APHIS Form 7002 provides a guideline for these situations and can be used for this purpose. A custom PVC can be created and used instead of this form if it covers all the aspects found within the APHIS Form 7002.[10]

As mentioned, the AV must have a formal arrangement with the regulated facility as either a full-time or part-time employee. It is important for the part-time AV to develop the PVC and record in writing all therapy and activities for the Animal Care Inspector to review. Full-time AVs can use their veterinary records. A schedule of regular visits for the part-time AV must be agreed on. The schedule is dictated by the nature of the facility and may be as few as once a year or twice monthly depending on need.[10]

The PVC must be updated whenever there is a change in AV, veterinary program, or veterinary practices. Any time a new species is added to the facility, the PVC must be updated to include that species. Chronic conditions of the animals, such as geriatric management, are optional for the AV to include in the PVC. At a minimum, the PVC should be updated annually, but more frequent updates may be necessary as determined by the AV[10] (**Box 2**).

Listed in **Figs. 2–6** are key parts of APHIS Form 7002. All parts of this form must be filled out entirely following the instructions as provided. Any similar format generated

---

Box 2
The program of veterinary care must

- Be in writing using either the APHIS Form 7002: Program of Veterinary Care for Research Facilities or Exhibitors/Dealers on page A-2, or a document containing equivalent information

- Address the following:
  - All covered species at the facility
  - Vaccinations (species, juveniles vs adults, list of vaccines, route schedule of when they are to be given, and whether they are to be given by the licensee or the AV)
  - Parasite control (ectoparasites, blood parasites, intestinal parasites, including required testing intervals, drugs to be used for prevention and treatment with ages of animals, dosages, route, and frequency)
  - Detailed description of emergency care availability and contact information
  - Detailed description of appropriate euthanasia to be used (personnel authorized to perform and the method)
  - Detailed description of capture and restraint method or methods. If more than one method is approved, there should be a detailed description of all approved method

- Address other topics pertinent to each licensee

- Be reviewed and updated as needed for situations, such as:
  - Change in the preventive medical program
  - New AV
  - Addition of a new species of animal
  - New location or site

- Be signed and dated by the AV and the licensee whenever it is changed, or reviewed without a change

- Include regularly scheduled visits to the licensee's facility frequently enough to provide adequate oversight

Data from United States Department of Agriculture (USDA). Animal Welfare Inspection Guide. USDA. 2013. Available at: https://www.aphis.usda.gov/animal_welfare/downloads/Animal-Care-Inspection-Guide.pdf. Accessed November 1, 2017.

must include, at a minimum, all aspects of this form. The complete APHIS Form 7002 is found online at: https://www.pdffiller.com/jsfiller-desk2/?projectId= 146576925&expId=2730&expBranch=1#b5ea02b6c4164f89bc2dcba13520f04e. The PDF fill-in is preferable to hand-written forms in the author's opinion.

REGULATED FACILITIES

AVs have the opportunity to help the licensee or registrant develop their care program for their animals. The AWA does not regulate the AV, only the facilities, which are inspected by the regional animal care inspector. The involvement of the AV ensures that the licensee, or registrant, is compliant with the PVC. Issues with noncompliance in relation to veterinary care are often due to a breakdown in communication between the licensee or registrant and the AV or failing to follow the PVC guidelines. The licensee or registrant is responsible for contacting the AV with any issues on animal health, behavior, and well-being.[1]

Animal care inspectors will make regular visits to the facility to review the PVC and the licensee or registrant's compliance. Any noncompliance found during inspection is referred to the facility and not the AV. AVs are encouraged to contact the USDA animal care inspector with any questions on their PVC. The facility itself is responsible for managing the PVC. Providing adequate facilities, personnel, equipment, and services to support the PVC are their responsibility. The animals must be observed daily with any signs of injury, disease, or behavior change being reported to the AV. Adequate record keeping is mandatory and should include animal observation and treatment logs, enrichment logs, vaccination and preventative health records, room maintenance logs, and standard operating procedures if available.[1] **Box 3** is a comprehensive list of the records the licensee or registrant must maintain taken from the USDA/APHIS Animal Care Guide[1] (see **Box 3**; **Boxes 4** and **5**).

According to the Paperwork Reduction Act of 1995, an agency may not conduct or sponsor, and a person is not required to respond to, a collection of information unless it displays a valid OMB control number. The valid OMB control numbers for these information collections are 0579-0036, 0579-0093, and 0579-0392. The time required to complete these information collections is estimated to average 1 hour per response, including the time for reviewing instructions, searching existing data sources, gathering and maintaining the data needed, and completing and reviewing the collection of information.

OMB Approved
0579-0036
0579-0093
0579-0392

The Animal Welfare Regulations, Title 9, Subchapter A, Part II, Subpart C, Section 2.33 and Subpart D, Section 2.40 require a Program of Veterinary Care.

UNITED STATES DEPARTMENT OF AGRICULTURE
ANIMAL AND PLANT HEALTH INSPECTION SERVICE

ANIMAL CARE
(Program of Veterinary Care for Research Facilities or Exhibitors/Dealers)

OFFICE USE ONLY
DATE RECEIVED:

SECTION I. A PROGRAM OF VETERINARY CARE HAS BEEN ESTABLISHED BETWEEN:

A. LICENSEE/REGISTRANT	B. VETERINARIAN
1. NAME:	1. NAME:
2. BUSINESS NAME:	2. CLINIC NAME:
3. USDA LICENSE/REGISTRATION NUMBER:	3. STATE LICENSE NUMBER:
4. MAILING ADDRESS:	4. BUSINESS ADDRESS:
5. CITY, STATE, AND ZIP CODE:	5. CITY, STATE, AND ZIP CODE:
6. TELEPHONE NUMBER *(Home):* TELEPHONE NUMBER *(Business):*	6. TELEPHONE NUMBER *(Business):*

Fig. 2. The first page of the form contains the client and veterinarian information. This area should be filled in, including the Coding Accuracy Support System-certified address for both the client and the veterinarian.

This is a form that may be used for the Program of Veterinary Care. Also, this form may be used as a guideline for the written Program of Veterinary Care, as required.

The attending veterinarian shall establish, maintain, and supervise programs of disease control and prevention, pest and parasite control, pre-procedural and post-procedural care, nutrition, euthanasia, and adequate veterinary care for all animals on the premises of the licensee/registrant.   A written program of adequate veterinary care between the licensee/registrant and the doctor of veterinary medicine shall be established and reviewed on an annual basis. By law, such programs must include regularly scheduled visits to the premises by the veterinarian. Scheduled visits are required to monitor animal health and husbandry.

Pages or blocks which do not apply to the facility should be marked N/A. If the space provided is not adequate for a specific topic, additional sheets may be added. Please indicate Section and Item Number.

I have read and completed this Program of Veterinary Care, and understand my responsibilities.

Regularly scheduled visits by the veterinarian will occur at the following frequency:

_____ (minimum annual).

C. SIGNATURE OF LICENSEE/REGISTRANT:	DATE:
D. SIGNATURE OF VETERINARIAN:	DATE:

APHIS 7002
JUN 2011

Page 1 of 4

Fig. 3. The formal agreement between the AV and the licensee or registrant. Number of minimum visits will need to be agreed on before you get to this page. Both signatures and both dates are needed.

Each marine mammal (MM) must have its own individual record kept where it is housed and available for APHIS inspection. If it is transferred to another facility, including contract and satellite facility, a copy of the health record must accompany it[1] (**Box 6**).

The PVC must be clear on the care of injuries, treatment of disease, vaccines administered, prescription medicine, parasites and pest control, nutrition, and reproduction for the facility. The facility must provide appropriate space for the AV to provide this care. The facility must also provide personnel with adequate training to carry out the prescribed therapy, handle the animals, manage wounds, attend to surgical

CHECK IF N/A ☐	SECTION III. WILD AND EXOTIC ANIMALS
A. VACCINATIONS – LIST THE DISEASES FOR WHICH VACCINATIONS ARE PERFORMED AND THE FREQUENCY OF THE VACCINATIONS *(Enter N/A if not applicable)*:	
CARNIVORES:	
HOOFED STOCK:	
PRIMATES:	
ELEPHANTS:	
MARINE MAMMALS:	
OTHER *(Specify)*:	

B. PARASITE CONTROL PROGRAM DESCRIBE THE FREQUENCY OF SAMPLING OR TREATMENT FOR THE FOLLOWING:

Fig. 4. The animals you are working with will be on page 3. Common names as well as genus and species are needed here. There is more space for additional animal descriptions on page 4 of the form.

B. PARASITE CONTROL PROGRAM – DESCRIBE THE FREQUENCY OF SAMPLING OR TREATMENT FOR THE FOLLOWING:

1. ECTOPARASITES *(Fleas, Ticks, Mites, Lice, Flies)*:

2. BLOOD PARASITES:

3. INTESTINAL PARASITES:

C. EMERGENCY CARE

1. DESCRIBE PROVISIONS FOR EMERGENCY, WEEKEND, AND HOLIDAY CARE:

2. DESCRIBE CAPTURE AND RESTRAINT METHOD(S):

D. EUTHANASIA

1. SICK, DISEASED, INJURED, OR LAME ANIMALS SHALL BE PROVIDED WITH VETERINARY CARE OR EUTHANIZED. EUTHANASIA WILL BE IN ACCORDANCE WITH THE AVMA RECOMMENDATIONS AND WILL BE CARRIED OUT BY THE FOLLOWING:

☐ VETERINARIAN   ☐ LICENSEE/REGISTRANT

2. METHOD(S) OF EUTHANASIA:

E. ADDITIONAL PROGRAM TOPICS – THE FOLLOWING TOPICS HAVE BEEN DISCUSSED IN THE FORMULATION OF THE PROGRAM OF VETERINARY CARE:

☐ Pest Control and Product Safety   ☐ Environment Enhancement *(Primates)*

☐ Quarantine Procedures   ☐ Water Quality *(Marine Mammals)*

☐ Zoonoses   ☐ Species-specific Behaviors

☐ Other *(Specify)* _____   ☐ Proper Storage and Handling of Drugs and Biologics

   _____   ☐ Proper Use of Analgesics and Sedatives

F. LIST THE SPECIES SUBJECTED TO TB TESTING, AND THE FREQUENCY OF SUCH TESTS:

APHIS 7002
JUN 2011   Page 3 of 4

Fig. 5. Part of the PVC on page 3 of the form. Provide succinct details here. A more formal PVC can be produced and attached as needed.

recovery, and euthanize animals where this task can be performed by someone who is not a veterinarian as allowed by state and local law. Proper care should be taken to adhere to the guidelines set down by the American Veterinary Medical Association and the American Association of Zoo Veterinarians[11] (**Box 7**).

CHECK IF N/A ☐   **SECTION IV. OTHER WARMBLOODED ANIMALS**

A. INDICATE SPECIES:

B. VACCINATIONS – LIST THE DISEASES FOR WHICH VACCINATIONS ARE PERFORMED AND THE FREQUENCY OF VACCINATIONS *(Enter N/A if not applicable)*:

C. PARASITE CONTROL PROGRAM – DESCRIBE THE FREQUENCY OF SAMPLING OR TREATMENT FOR THE FOLLOWING:

1. ECTOPARASITES *(Fleas, Ticks, Mites, Lice, Flies)*:

2. INTERNAL PARASITES *(Helminths, Coccidia, Other)*:

Fig. 6. Page 4 provides space for listing additional animals. Common names as well as genus and species will be needed.

Box 3
Recommended records: a licensee/registrant should maintain the following records to demonstrate that he/she is providing an adequate program of veterinary care, when applicable

- Animal observation and treatment logs, which could include:
  - Documentation of an acute or chronic medical issue
  - Documentation of contact with the AV
  - Treatment prescribed by the AV
  - Treatment records, that is, dates and times of treatment if applicable
  - Results of treatment

- AV approval of noncommercial diet for large felids

- Feeding of young animals, such as bottle feeding

- Vaccination and preventive health records (individual animal or group/litter)

- Necropsy records

- Surgery records

- Euthanasia records

- Cage wash validation sheets

- Room maintenance logs

- Standard operating procedures, if available

- Acclimation statements for transportation

- AV-approved exemptions

- Written PVC for part-time or consulting AV

Data from United States Department of Agriculture (USDA). Animal Welfare Inspection Guide. USDA. 2013. Available at: https://www.aphis.usda.gov/animal_welfare/downloads/Animal-Care-Inspection-Guide.pdf. Accessed November 1, 2017.

Box 4
Recommended records for nonhuman primates: in addition to the required records listed in Box 3, the following records requiring veterinary approval are required for nonhuman primates, when applicable

- Environmental enhancement plan

- Health certificates for transport

- Approval for acclimation to higher temperatures for
  - Sheltered housing
  - Outdoor housing
  - Mobile/traveling housing

- Humidity levels for:
  - Indoor housing
  - Sheltered housing

- AV-approved exemptions

Data from United States Department of Agriculture (USDA). Animal Welfare Inspection Guide. USDA. 2013. Available at: https://www.aphis.usda.gov/animal_welfare/downloads/Animal-Care-Inspection-Guide.pdf. Accessed November 1, 2017.

Box 5
Recommended records for marine mammals

In addition to the required records listed in **Box 3**, the following records requiring veterinary approval are required for MMs, when applicable:

- Health certificates for transport
- Individual MM medical records
- Necropsy records

Individual MM medical records must be kept and include the following information, at a minimum:

- Animal identification/name
- A physical description, such as:
- Identifying markings
  ○ Scars
  ○ Age
  ○ Sex
- Physical examination information including, but not limited to:
  ○ All diagnostic test results
  ○ Documentation of treatment
  ○ Identification of all medical and physical problems
  ○ Length
  ○ Physical examination results by body system
  ○ Proposed plan of action for medical/physical problems
  ○ Weight
- Visual examination information

Data from United States Department of Agriculture (USDA). Animal Welfare Inspection Guide. USDA. 2013. Available at: https://www.aphis.usda.gov/animal_welfare/downloads/Animal-Care-Inspection-Guide.pdf. Accessed November 1, 2017.

Box 6
Recommended records for marine mammal necropsy reports

The preliminary necropsy report must:

- Be prepared by the veterinarian conducting the necropsy
- List all pathologic lesions observed

The final necropsy report must include:

- All gross findings
- All histopathology findings
- A pathologic diagnosis
- Results of all laboratory tests performed

Necropsy reports must be:

- Available for APHIS inspection
- Kept for 3 years
- Maintained at the home facility of the MM, AND
- Maintained at the facility where the MM died, if different than the home facility

Data from United States Department of Agriculture (USDA). Animal Welfare Inspection Guide. USDA. 2013. Available at: https://www.aphis.usda.gov/animal_welfare/downloads/Animal-Care-Inspection-Guide.pdf. Accessed November 1, 2017.

Box 7
Acceptable methods of euthanasia

The method of euthanasia should be evaluated to ensure that:

- It is listed as an acceptable method of euthanasia in the AVMA Euthanasia Guidelines

- If the method is designated in the AVMA Guidelines as acceptable "with conditions," ensure that the conditions have been met and are fully described in the PVC

- The person performing the euthanasia, if not a veterinarian, is qualified and has the proper training

Data from United States Department of Agriculture (USDA). Animal Welfare Inspection Guide. USDA. 2013. Available at: https://www.aphis.usda.gov/animal_welfare/downloads/Animal-Care-Inspection-Guide.pdf. Accessed November 1, 2017.

The facility's veterinary records must be kept for at least 1 year after the animal's disposition or death or as required by APHIS, or longer, if required by other applicable laws or policies.[1] These records must be readily available at all times for the APHIS officials to review. These records may also remain at the AV's veterinary clinic but must be available upon request.

Certain exotics have detailed requirements of care and authorization. Keeping a close eye on the amendments to the AWA and the Animal Welfare Inspection Guide are key.[12,13]

NONHUMAN PRIMATES AND MARINE MAMMALS

Health certificates with the signature of the AV will be necessary on all nonhuman primates (NHPs) that are transported interstate, in foreign commerce, and intrastate by commercial carriers (**Boxes 8** and **9**). The AV will also need a signature accompanying all MM necropsy reports, health certificates for transport of MMs, and temperature acclimation certificates for transport of MMs.[1]

REGULATED RESEARCH FACILITIES

The same formal agreement must exist between the full- or part-time AV and the research facility as occurs with the previously discussed facilities. The AV will also need to work closely with the Institutional Care and Use Committee (IACUC) to ensure adequate veterinary care and oversight of the animals occurs. Guidance to the principle investigators is provided by the AV and includes handling, immobilization, anesthesia, analgesia, tranquilization, and euthanasia. All aspects of surgery including preprocedural and postprocedural care must be managed in line with current veterinary standards.

The IACUC consists of at least 3 people, one of which must be a veterinarian, often the AV. It exists to review the research facility's procedures, facilities, and animal program. It is required for evaluating the care, treatment, use of animals, and housing provided. The IACUC is necessary for certifying compliance with the AWA by the research facility. Every 6 months or more often, the IACUC reviews key elements of care. These elements of care include the facility's program for humane care and use of animals. They also inspect animal facilities, prepare reports, and investigate complaints as they occur.[1,2,10]

Only qualified individuals as listed in **Box 10** can be IACUC members so that they can properly assess the research facility's animal program, facilities, and procedures. The responsibility lies with the research facility for ensuring their qualification. The training and instruction will be provided by the facility and should include the AWA, protocol review, and facility inspections[10] (see **Box 10**).

Box 8

In nonhuman primates, the approval of the attending veterinarian is required for the following

- Ambient temperature of indoor housing and the sheltered portion of sheltered housing facilities for NHPs
- Relative humidity level of indoor housing and the sheltered portion of sheltered housing facilities for NHPs
- Outdoor housing of NHPs
- Outdoor housing of NHPs with shelters that do not provide heat to prevent the ambient temperature from falling below 45°F
- Ambient temperature in mobile or traveling housing facilities for NHP
- Environmental enhancement plan for NHPs, including AV approvals for:
  ○ Social grouping
  ○ Isolation of NHPs that have or are suspected of having a contagious disease
  ○ Determination of compatibility of NHPs for social housing
  ○ Approval of singly housed NHPs to not be able to see/hear other NHPs
  ○ Special considerations for NHPs requiring special attention, including:
    ■ Infants and young juveniles
    ■ NHPs showing signs of psychological distress
    ■ Individually housed NHPs that cannot see/hear their own or compatible species
    ■ Great apes weighing more than 50 kg
- Maintenance of NHPs in restraint devices for health reasons
- Statements of exemptions from participation in the environmental enhancement plan for individual NHPs
- Restriction of water for NHPs
  ○ Approval of no food or water for NHPs during transport by a carrier or intermediate handler

Data from United States Department of Agriculture (USDA). Animal Welfare Inspection Guide. USDA. 2013. Available at: https://www.aphis.usda.gov/animal_welfare/downloads/Animal-Care-Inspection-Guide.pdf. Accessed November 1, 2017.

Box 9

In marine mammals, the approval of the attending veterinarian is required for the following

- Statement of exemptions to MM housing requirements, including:
  ○ Housing in smaller than required enclosures for nonmedical training, breeding, or holding for more than 2 weeks
  ○ Housing in smaller than required enclosures for transfer for more than 1 week
- Feeding MM less than once per day
- Application of insecticides and other such chemical agents in primary enclosures housing MM
- Approval for the single housing of social MM
- Approval to house newly acquired MM with resident animals
- Holding of MM in a medical treatment or medical training enclosure that does not meet the minimum space requirements for more than 2 weeks
- Procedure for cleaning and/or sanitizing an enclosure that has housed an MM with an infectious or contagious disease
- Frequency of feeding for an MM in transit
- Transport plan for transport of an MM lasting more than 2 hours in duration

Data from United States Department of Agriculture (USDA). Animal Welfare Inspection Guide. USDA. 2013. Available at: https://www.aphis.usda.gov/animal_welfare/downloads/Animal-Care-Inspection-Guide.pdf. Accessed November 1, 2017.

Box 10
Qualification requirements to be a veterinary member of an Institutional Care and Use Committee

- Ability to critically review a protocol for veterinary care issues, and

- Direct or delegated authority for activities involving animals at the research facility, and

- Training or experience in laboratory animal science and medicine

- A research facility's AV may fulfill the role of the DVM on the IACUC, or the position may be filled by another veterinarian.

Data from United States Department of Agriculture (USDA). Animal Welfare Inspection Guide. USDA. 2013. Available at: https://www.aphis.usda.gov/animal_welfare/downloads/Animal-Care-Inspection-Guide.pdf. Accessed November 1, 2017.

Box 11
Supplemental information and materials

Audio tapes provided by the research facility

Cage wash water temperature certification records

E-mails and e-mail records

IACUC facility inspection reports

IACUC-related correspondence

Interviews with IACUC members

Maintenance records

Medical/surgical records

Memos and notes

Program of humane care and use

Room temperature logs

Standard operating procedures

Written meeting minutes

Data from United States Department of Agriculture (USDA). Animal Welfare Inspection Guide. USDA. 2013. Available at: https://www.aphis.usda.gov/animal_welfare/downloads/Animal-Care-Inspection-Guide.pdf. Accessed November 1, 2017.

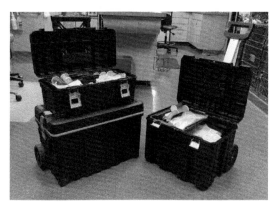

Fig. 7. Rolling tool cases make it easy to be organized outside of the hospital. Pictured are 2 multicompartment mobile cart/toolboxes that are ideal for transporting small equipment and supplies.

The information in **Box 11** represents supplemental information and materials that the facility can provide that can help verify or assess IACUC function and will be necessary for the Animal Care Inspector to review. Documents that will be reviewed to assess IACUC function may include, but are *not* limited to the following.

Equipment and Supplies

Being prepared for your facility's visit is very much like being prepared for a house call. Take into consideration the type of visit planned and pack accordingly. If this is an annual visit, prepare to bring along equipment necessary for sampling and

---

Box 12
Recommended equipment

The following equipment is highly recommended:

- Examination forms, clipboard
- Pen/pencil
- Thermometer or temperature gun
- Scale that measures in grams
- Nitrile gloves
- Syringes, needles, blood collection vials
- Alcohol, gauze pads
- Slides, coverslips, saline, safe transport container
- Culturettes, copan swabs, sterile cotton tip applicators
- Stethoscope
- Disposable booties, caps, masks, sterile gloves
- Bandage material
- Emergency kit
- Disinfectant/soap
- Tape measure
- Calculator
- Absorbent pads

The following items are suggested

- Ear plugs
- Towels, paper towels
- Flash light and extra batteries
- Note pad

The following items are optional

- Microscope
- General surgical pack
- Extra scrubs or isolation gown
- Business cards
- Camera/cell phone
- Laptop computer

Box 13
Special equipment for macaques, nonhuman primates, and elephants

The following equipment is recommended for inspecting facilities with macaques, if within 5 feet of the macaques:

- Biological waste bag
- Isolation gown, cap, gloves
- Disinfectant
- Disposable gloves
- Exposure kit
- Full face shield and eye protection, such as safety glasses or goggles
- Respirator

The following equipment is recommended for inspecting facilities with other NHPs and elephants:

- Respirator: Level N95 or better

---

vaccinating. Having a well-trained technician or assistant is equally important. The additional professional help ensures quality teamwork and improves the efficiency of the visit. The facility must provide a clean space to accomplish the visit and examine the animals. Much of the equipment is in place already. Good communications with the facility before the visit should delineate what equipment is needed for the visit. Transporting the equipment will require that you find a sturdy toolbox or equivalent on wheels. The author prefers the 2 box types to be the handiest (**Fig. 7**). **Boxes 12** and **13** feature a general checklist of equipment to consider.

SUMMARY

Exotic veterinarians can enjoy the benefits of being an AV for a USDA/APHIS regulated facility by expanding their normal day to include interesting species and locations. Participating in keeping these animals healthy and well cared for is satisfying and rewarding. Being familiar with the AWA and The Animal Care Policy Manual produced by the USDA/APHIS is an important part of the job. Creating a PVC either using USDA Form 7002 or expanding this form to a customized format is an integral part of the exotic veterinarian's contribution to the facility. Understanding the function of the IACUC is an important aspect of being an AV for a research facility.

REFERENCES

1. USDA APHIS | animal care and inspection Guide. USDA/APHIS; 2013. Available at: https://www.aphis.usda.gov/animal_welfare/downloads/Animal-Care-Inspection-Guide.pdf. Accessed November 1, 2017.
2. USDA APHIS | Animal Welfare Act. USDA/APHIS; 2017. Available at: https://www.aphis.usda.gov/animal_welfare/downloads/AC_BlueBook_AWA_FINAL_2017_508comp.pdf. Accessed November 1, 2017.
3. The Animal Welfare Act. Cohen, Henry. 12, s.l. Michigan State University of Law; 2006. Vol. Journal of Animal Law.
4. USDA APHIS | veterinary accreditation. USDA/APHIS; 2017. Available at: https://www.aphis.usda.gov/aphis/ourfocus/animalhealth/nvap/ct_add_info. Accessed January 29, 2018.

5. USDA APHIS | 9 CFR Parts 160, 161, and 162 NVAP Final Rule. USDA APHIS. Available at: https://www.aphis.usda.gov/animal_health/vet_accreditation/downloads/CFR_Parts_160-161-162.pdf. Accessed January 29, 2018.

6. Association, California Veterinary Medical. Update on veterinary accreditation. California Veterinary Medical Association. Available at: https://cvma.net/government/regulatory-and-cal-osha/health-certificates-airline-transportation-information/national-veterinary-accreditation-program/. Accessed January 29, 2018.

7. USDA APHIS | VS Form 1–36A. USDA/APHIS. Available at: https://www.aphis.usda.gov/animal_health/vet_accreditation/downloads/vs1-36a.pdf. Accessed January 29, 2018.

8. USDA APHIS | AWA program. USDA/APHIS; 2017. Available at: https://www.aphis.usda.gov/aphis/ourfocus/animalwelfare/sa_awa/ct_awa_program_information.

9. RACE. AAVSB RACE. Available at: https://www.aavsb.org/RACE/. Accessed February 9, 2018.

10. USDA APHIS | animal care manual. USDA APHIS; 2017. Available at: https://www.aphis.usda.gov/animal_welfare/downloads/Animal%20Care%20Policy%20Manual.pdf.

11. Leary S, Underwood W, Eli Lilly and Company, et al. AVMA guidelines for the Euthanasia of animals. AVMA Policies; 2013. Available at: https://www.avma.org/KB/Policies/Documents/euthanasia.pdf. Accessed February 14, 2018.

12. AAZV Euthanasia guidelines. Available at: http://www.aazv.org/?441. Accessed January 29, 2018.

13. USDA APHIS | Updates to AWA page. USDA APHIS; 2017. Available at: https://content.govdelivery.com/accounts/USDAAPHIS/bulletins/184e0d0. Accessed February 14, 2018.

Ambulatory Zoo Practice

David Hannon, DVM, DABVP (Avian)

KEYWORDS

• Ambulatory • Zoo • Mobile • Field • Anesthesia

KEY POINTS

- Ambulatory zoologic practice carries many challenges due to myriad species that may need veterinary care; therefore, proper preparedness is key.
- The necessary equipment, medications, and supplies should either accompany the veterinarian or be available at the site where the work is performed.
- Knowledge of the care and feeding of these animals and the legalities of owning and working with them is imperative.
- Being able to address medical and surgical issues in a field setting is a necessary skill for the ambulatory zoo veterinarian to master.

INTRODUCTION

Because of myriad species that may be seen in a zoologic setting, proper preparedness for the veterinary needs of these animals is imperative. The veterinary care of aquatic, avian, and herpetological species in a zoologic setting is similar, with the possible exception of ratites, storks and cranes, giant tortoises, crocodilians, larger fish species (eg, sharks and rays), and the like. This article primarily focuses on the veterinary care of exotic mammals that may be found in a zoologic setting.

THE CLIENT

Most large zoos, safari parks, aquariums, and animal theme parks and, even some private collections have resident veterinarians and designated veterinary facilities to provide medical and surgical care for their animals. Some smaller zoos, however, even if publicly owned, may not have neither the collection size nor budget to warrant employing a full-time veterinarian. These zoos often contract with a local veterinarian to provide services either on a regular or as-needed basis. Privately owned collections of nontraditional species also tend to operate in this manner. Some traditional farms may branch out into exotic animals, and there are also situations where an individual chooses to own a small number of exotic animals that cannot be practically

Disclosure Statement: This author has nothing to disclose.
Avian and Exotic Animal Veterinary Services, PetVax Complete Care Centers, 3650 Southwind Park Cove, Memphis, TN 38125, USA
E-mail address: hannondvm@msn.com

Vet Clin Exot Anim 21 (2018) 685–697
https://doi.org/10.1016/j.cvex.2018.05.005
1094-9194/18/© 2018 Elsevier Inc. All rights reserved.

transported to a veterinarian when care is needed. The author has clients who use a local veterinarian for routine work for the more common species kept and then contact the author if specialized care is needed for the more unique species.

THE BUSINESS

Veterinarians who have zoologic experience, are board certified (ie, American College of Zoological Medicine (ACZM), European College of Zoological Medicine (ECZM), or American Board of Veterinary Practitioners (ABVP)), or work in practices with a reputation for dealing with nontraditional species may be approached by a zoologic collection owner or manager who needs their services, particularly if they advertise themselves as such. Practitioners who are just starting out in the field of zoologic medicine and surgery may want to reach out to local zoologic facilities directly and offer their services. If veterinarians are inexperienced with the species that a local zoo keeps, they may want to offer to volunteer their time to learn about those species, because it may open a door for future gainful employment.

To stay in business, veterinarians must charge appropriately for their services; this also holds true for ambulatory zoo veterinarians. The owners of a collection should be informed of these fees up front so they are prepared to pay for a veterinarian's services. There are many different fee structures and methods of billing, but the author's practice reflects that of a traditional ambulatory food animal practice. This includes a travel charge that is billed per mile 1 way and an hourly rate billed in 15-minute increments, with a 1-hour minimum. This fee covers all services that are performed on site, including examinations, sample collection, professional services (such as hoof trims and wound care), surgery, and necropsy. The client is billed an additional amount for drugs and supplies that are used from the veterinarian's inventory, an equipment use fee for certain specialized equipment that the veterinarian owns, and the cost of any diagnostic testing that is performed off site. Fees should reflect the veterinarian's experience and expertise and be adequate to cover the cost of services and goods sold with a reasonable profit. Ideally, fees should be collected at the time services are rendered, but clients can be billed if they have a good relationship with the veterinarian or practice. Some ambulatory zoo practitioners charge a flat monthly rate that covers certain tasks and visits or are paid on a retainer basis to be available as needed.

NECESSARY EQUIPMENT AND SUPPLIES

Ambulatory zoo practice mimics ambulatory farm call practice in many ways, and a mobile zoo practitioner can be outfitted similarly. If an individual veterinarian is responsible for providing services for several smaller collections, then having an appropriate vehicle that is properly stocked with needed materials is often necessary. If a veterinarian is only servicing 1 or 2 collections, however, particularly if they are larger collections, then the veterinarian may consider working with the collection owner or manager to have the necessary equipment available on site. The veterinarian may also want to visit the collection for a consult prior to performing any veterinary services to determine which supplies and equipment are available or needed and to make sure that work areas are conducive to the work that needs to be performed.

- Vehicle: a veterinarian whose practice is primarily ambulatory may want to invest in a vehicle that is suited for this type of practice. There are specific trucks, truck inserts, vans, and recreational vehicle (RV)–type vehicles that are commercially available and may be appropriate for this kind of work. For traditional clinic-bound veterinarians who are branching out into ambulatory practice, however, this type of purchase can often not be financially justified. Often a suitable truck or sport utility vehicle may be adaptable to the needs of the ambulatory practitioner, and there have been many ambulatory veterinarians who have successfully practiced out of sedans and hatchbacks. Depending on the location, the size of the collection, and the type of facility, 4-wheel drive vehicles may be necessary to access certain areas. Most collections have appropriate vehicles for traversing their facility, and the use of their vehicles may be warranted, but this entails transferring the necessary equipment and supplies. Having access to a trailer that is suitable for transporting larger species may be beneficial if an animal has to be translocated out of the collection to an isolated pen, stall, or veterinary facility.

- Equipment: the type of equipment needed depends on the species being treated. For collections that are primarily hoofstock, the same equipment used for ambulatory food animal and equine practice is often necessary. Great apes may require human medical equipment. For carnivores, smaller primates, and other similar-sized species, equipment for companion animal practice may be adequate. For small species, such as rodents or bats, more specialized equipment may be needed, such as magnification and microsurgical instrumentation (**Table 1**).
- Supplies: the supplies needed often vary with the different species that are being treated. Some items, like vaccinations or tuberculin, are species-specific, whereas certain antibiotics and other medications or items may be usable across a broad range of species. For items that are more unique and species-specific, particularly if they are only available in larger quantities, such as vaccines, the collection owner or manager should be encouraged to purchase the entire batch for specific use with only their animals (**Table 2**).

LEGAL RAMIFICATIONS

There are many legal issues that an ambulatory practitioner needs to be aware of. There are certain ones, however, that a zoologic practitioner needs to be made aware of (**Table 3**).

QUARANTINE AND ISOLATION

As per the American Association of Zoo Veterinarians "Guidelines for Zoo and Aquarium Veterinary Medical Programs and Veterinary Hospitals,"[2] new arrivals to a facility should ideally be quarantined separate from the rest of the collection for a minimum period of 30 days, or longer, depending on the species. Although not all private zoos and collections adhere to this policy, the veterinarian consulting for the collection should encourage this practice. Animals in quarantine should have a physical or visual examination on entering and leaving quarantine, with appropriate diagnostic testing performed during the stay to assure that the animal is healthy and to help prevent the introduction of new diseases into the collection. Many facilities request that diagnostic testing of this nature be performed by the originating institution prior to shipping the animal(s).

Animals that are sick or injured often need to be removed from the collection to prevent the transmission of infectious agents or trauma from conspecifics, or to prevent self-trauma and facilitate return to function. Isolation areas should be just that, isolated from the rest of the collection and from the public, and ideally from other isolated animals. These animals need to be assessed by the veterinarian on a frequent basis and

Table 1
The type of equipment needed depends on the species being treated

Capture equipment	• Remote drug delivery systems (ie, dart guns, blow guns, etc.; see text) may be needed for larger animals or animals housed in large exhibits. • Gloves, nets, catchpoles, pole syringes, and the like may be more suitable for smaller species in smaller enclosures. • Squeeze cages, stocks, and cattle chutes can also be beneficial, but these items ideally should be available at the facility because they are often not readily portable. • For larger animals, halters and ropes are handy to aid in restraint and positioning after an animal has been sedated. • Transport cages, such as dog crates, may also be needed to transport smaller animals to another area or to a veterinary facility. • Minimizing stress to an animal during capture and restraint is important to prevent morbidity.
Diagnostic equipment	• Smaller instruments, such as microscopes, centrifuges, thermometers, refractometers, and pulse oximeters, are easily transported and can be readily used on site. • Imaging equipment (portable x-ray and ultrasound) and laboratory analyzers are more difficult to transport and use in the field, but they offer the benefit of a quicker diagnosis. • Stethoscopes, otoscopes, and ophthalmoscopes are necessary for a complete physical examination. • A good pair of binoculars is always warranted to aid in the evaluation of animals from a distance.
Surgical equipment	• Having the appropriate instrumentation available for surgical procedures is important. Just because a surgery may be taking place in the field, a barn, the back of a truck, or on a kitchen table, adherence to proper instrument sterilization and aseptic surgical technique is still the best standard of care. • Surgical instruments should ideally be properly wrapped and sterilized prior to the visit, and cold sterilization should be available if needed. • For invasive procedures, caps, masks, and sterile gowns, gloves, and drapes should be available.
Dental equipment	• Dental health is an important aspect of zoologic medicine, and thoroughly evaluating the mouth of animals when an opportunity arises is warranted. • Having equipment available for floating teeth, tooth scaling and polishing, probing, and tooth extraction is necessary to maintain good oral health.
Foot, hoof, horn, and antler care equipment	• Foot and hoof issues occur commonly in captive exotic ungulates and can be associated with being housed on a substrate that may be unsuitable for their species. • Fractured horns and antlers can occur when animals fight or run into barriers. In cervid collections, antlers often must be selectively removed to prevent fighting for dominance. • When working with these species, hoof trimmers, hoof knives, saws, nail trimmers, and cauterization equipment are a must. • Some facilities may contract with farriers for some of these services.

(continued on next page)

Table 1 (continued)	
Animal identification equipment	• Being able to identify individual animals within a collection is important for proper record keeping and case management. • Although most zoologic collections are moving toward using microchips and passive integrated transponder (PIT) tags, there are some that still use ear tags, ear notching, tattoos, and brands. • The means of animal identification should be discussed with the collection owner or manager prior to any usage. • Potentially painful procedures should ideally be performed under general anesthesia.
Necropsy equipment	• Equipment used for animal necropsy should ideally be limited for use in that capacity. Using procedural or surgical equipment to perform necropsies may result in damage or contamination to these instruments. • Necropsy knives, saws, rib cutters, and the like should be available and kept sanitized.
Personal protective gear	• Many of the animals that are kept in zoologic collections are inherently dangerous, and protecting oneself from injury and zoonoses is critical. Protective head gear, eye protection, hearing protection, gloves, boots, and the like should be available if needed.
Administrative equipment	• Laptop computers, pads, and smartphones are an essential part of ambulatory practice in today's digital era. • Medical record keeping, invoicing, inventory, managing laboratory results and digital images, and fee collection are just as important to the ambulatory practitioner as they are to the brick-and-mortar practice. • Smartphones and tablets have made it simple to create invoices and collect fees on site where services are rendered.

should be cleared by the veterinarian prior to their introduction or return to the collection.

REMOTE AND FIELD ANESTHESIA

Sedation, anesthesia, and anxiolytic medications are often necessary to reduce pain or distress when working with zoologic species. Physical restraint without sedation should be used only for brief noninvasive procedures in individual animals that are appropriate for manual restraint. Animals that are kept in small enclosures, have night houses, or have been trained by operant conditioning often can be directly immobilized with minimal distress and effort. Animals that are free range, kept in larger enclosures, or are unconditioned to humans, however, often require remote immobilization. In a smaller enclosure, hand injections, syringe poles, and blowguns work well for close-range situations, but in larger enclosures or in the field, a projectile dart is often necessary to immobilize an animal. The ambulatory zoo veterinarian should be well versed in the drugs and delivery systems used in these scenarios. Training can be obtained through Safe-Capture International (www.safecapture.com) or other similar programs. There are many resources for drug selection and dosing for the species being immobilized.[3–6] Controlled substances should be maintained according to Drug Enforcement Administration (DEA) guidelines.[7] If controlled substances are kept at the facility for emergency use when the veterinarian is not present (eg, the escape

Table 2
The supplies needed often vary with the different species that are being treated

Medications	• Some medications, such as broad-spectrum antibiotics, anti-inflammatories, crystalloid fluids, and narcotic analgesics, have a broad range of doses and can be used across several different species. • Injectable medications are most often used in zoologic collections, but sometimes oral medications are also necessary. These may be more difficult to stock because there is a lot of variability in the strength and formulations needed. Relationships with nearby veterinary practices and pharmacies aid in supplying these medications when needed. • Because exotic animals can be difficult to medicate, long-acting formulations are useful in increasing compliance and decreasing animal stress. • All prescription medications, not just controlled substances, should be kept in a designated area and only be used by or on the order of the veterinarian. • If any of the animals in the collection are used to produce meat, milk, or eggs for human consumption, proper withdrawal times should be followed (www.farad.org).
Surgical supplies	• Sterile surgery blades, suture material, drapes, gowns, and the like should be on hand for needed surgical procedures. These are most often going to be used for simple procedures, such as wound repair or castration, but veterinarians must be prepared for more invasive procedures, such as enucleations, amputations, or cesarean sections. • More involved surgeries, such as orthopedic procedures or exploratory laparotomies, should ideally be planned well in advance so that the necessary equipment and supplies are available.
Sundries	• Syringes, gauze, cotton, bandage material, examination gloves, and so forth should all be stocked and accessible when needed. • Rubbing alcohol, hydrogen peroxide, and disinfection scrubs and solutions, such as chlorhexidine or betadine, should also be readily available and stored in easily transported spill-proof containers.
Laboratory supplies	• If samples are being collected for laboratory analysis, then blood collection tubes, specimen containers, slides, cover slips, fecal containers, formalin jars, culture swabs, and the like should all be stocked and ready for use. • If diagnostic testing is being performed on site, then having the appropriate stains, fecal float solution, analyzer supplies, and so forth is necessary.

of a dangerous animal), then the veterinarian needs to have a separate DEA license for that facility, the drugs should be kept in a secured area only accessible by individuals authorized with their use, proper controlled drug logs should be maintained, and the veterinarian should be notified immediately if controlled substances are to be used in their absence. The DEA license holder is ultimately responsible for the use and storage of these drugs and the DEA should be consulted for the specifics of applicable regulations.

Once an animal has been immobilized, the veterinarian and support staff should be well versed in maintaining and monitoring anesthesia, anesthesia reversal, and preventing injury to the animal and personnel. Portable anesthetic monitors, blood gas analyzers (eg, i-STAT [Abbott Laboratories, IL, USA]), and a good stethoscope are

Table 3	
There are many legal issues that the zoologic practitioner needs to be aware of	
The contract	• As ambulatory zoo practitioners, veterinarians should be assured of fair compensation for their services. • Whether a veterinarian is working as a private contractor, a practice employee, or an employee of the zoologic facility, the terms of the professional agreement should be spelled out on the front end. • A good contract should delineate fee structure, payment terms, veterinarian or practice compensation, the liability of both parties, insurance, licensure, who supplies what equipment and supplies, and whatever else is deemed appropriate. • This document should ideally be reviewed by the veterinarian's lawyer to assure that it is fair and equitable but also protects the veterinarian appropriately. • Individual veterinarians or practices that contract with several zoologic facilities might want to put together a standard contract to cover their needs, while making specific adjustments based on the needs of the facility.
DEA licensure	• According to the DEA, mobile veterinarians are registered at their base of operations and storage of controlled substances should be at the registered location. If controlled substances are to be kept at another location, then the veterinarian must be registered at both locations. • Mobile units should be stocked with only enough of each drug for basic operation, and excess supplies should remain in the registered location. If kept on the vehicle, controlled drugs should be locked in a secure compartment or box that is securely mounted to the vehicle. • More information can be found at www.dea.gov.
State licensure	• Ambulatory veterinarians who travel to collections that are out of their state of licensure should contact the board of veterinary examiners for that state that they are traveling to in order to determine what type of licensure they need. • Some states have license reciprocity with surrounding states, whereas others offer temporary licensure, or they may require full state licensure to practice in their state. • This topic should be researched prior to the first appointment, because there may be significant penalties or legal liabilities. • Contacting each state's veterinary board should yield the information needed.
USDA licensure	• According to the USDA, exhibitors (individuals or businesses with warm-blooded animals that are on display, are used in educational presentations, or perform for the public) must be licensed with the Animal and Plant Inspection Service (APHIS). These include circuses, zoos, educational displays, petting farms/zoos, animal acts, wildlife parks, marine mammal parks, and some sanctuaries. The animals involved in the exhibition may include domestic and exotic animal species. • The USDA animal care inspectors conduct routine, unannounced inspections of all entities licensed/registered under the Animal Welfare Act. • During routine inspections, the USDA reviews the premises, records, husbandry practices, program of veterinary care, and animal handling procedures to ensure the animals are receiving humane care. • These facilities must have a veterinary inspection annually, and the veterinarian is required to fill out with Animal and Plant Inspection Service Form 7002, Animal Care (Program of Veterinary Care for Research Facilities or Exhibitors/Dealers), which must be kept on file on

(continued on next page)

Table 3 (continued)	
	site. This form states that "The attending veterinarian shall establish, maintain, and supervise programs of disease control and prevention, pest and parasite control, pre-procedural and post-procedural care, nutrition, euthanasia, and adequate veterinary care for all animals on the premises of the licensee/registrant. A written program of adequate veterinary care between the licensee/registrant and the doctor of veterinary medicine shall be established and reviewed on an annual basis. By law, such programs must include regularly scheduled visits to the premises by the veterinarian. Scheduled visits are required to monitor animal health and husbandry."[1] • More information can be found at www.aphis.usda.gov/aphis/ourfocus/animalwelfare.
Animal shipping	• If animals are shipped from the collection either interstate or internationally, the veterinarian needs to be accredited by the USDA to write health certificates for these animals. • Information on veterinary accreditation and animal shipping can be found at www.aphis.usda.gov/aphis/ourfocus/animalhealth/nvap.
Professional liability and bailment insurance	• Having appropriate insurance coverage is absolutely necessary. Without legal protection, malpractice and property damage claims can be financially devastating. • Veterinarians should consult with their liability insurance provider to make sure they have adequate coverage should an event arise at a zoologic client's facility. • If veterinarians are using a personal vehicle for ambulatory practice, they should contact their automobile insurance provider to ensure that they are properly covered.

invaluable in this regard. Some animals, in particular larger ones, often perfuse poorly under general anesthesia, and oxygen supplementation should be available if needed. The veterinarian should be informed and prepared for the prevention and/or treatment of capture myopathy, respiratory or cardiac arrest, hyperthermia or hypothermia, and other emergency situations. The immobilized animal should be monitored closely during recovery. This is even more important in field anesthesia when there are other animals present. Recently immobilized animals are often unable to react appropriately to their conspecifics and are at risk to be injured or for injuring themselves or personnel on anesthesia recovery. Other animals should be kept at a distance while the immobilized animal recovers.

WORKING AREAS

Some zoologic facilities have designated working areas for veterinarians. These may include anything from a full veterinary facility to a simple room or stall in a barn. The ambulatory zoo veterinarian needs to be aware of the areas where they will be practicing and the equipment that is available so they can be prepared to provide the needed services. If an area has not been designated for this purpose, then the veterinarian often has to improvise. The author has performed many procedures on portable tables, the backs of trucks, or in the middle of an open field. Regardless of the location, the area should ideally be as clean as possible and care should be taken to maintain sterility or aseptic technique as much as is possible. No matter where the procedure is performed, organization is key to a successful outcome. If a facility wants to have the veterinarian to come out on a regular basis, it is wise to establish a designated working area at the facility that can be kept cleaned and stocked with equipment and supplies.

Most farms and many private zoos and safari parks have pens, chutes, and headgates suitable for managing cattle or other livestock. If exotic animals are to be managed in this setting, they should be acclimated to it to reduce stress and anxiety, and the equipment has to be appropriate for the animals being managed. For example, most cattle chutes cannot accommodate large horns or antlers and are often too large to safely use on smaller species, like deer or alpacas. When dealing with these species/concerns, attention to detail must be paid in advance of the procedure.

DIAGNOSTICS

Point-of-care diagnostics are beneficial in providing a rapid diagnosis and initiating appropriate treatments sooner. Delayed results may require a second immobilization or may delay appropriate treatment, putting an animal at further risk. Point-of-care diagnostics, however, are not always practical or available.

- Imaging: regular fixed x-ray or ultrasound units are only suitable for smaller animals or ones that are very well trained. Smaller portable x-ray or ultrasound units are more practical for ambulatory practice. Digital radiography provides the most rapid results, but portable digital radiography units are expensive and cumbersome. Computed radiography and traditional x-ray film tend to be more practical for use in the field, but both take time for processing images, and many models/brands cannot be processed in the field. Establishing a good technique chart is essential for acquiring good-quality diagnostic images and decreasing the need to repeat radiographs. Many small portable radiology and ultrasound units are now commercially available and reasonably priced.
- Laboratory testing: larger zoos and safari parks with veterinary facilities often have point-of-care blood cell counters and blood chemistry analyzers, but these are not practical for most smaller collections. There are mobile devices that can provide some of these data, such as the Abaxis VetScan [Abaxis Inc, CA, USA] or the i-STAT, that the ambulatory zoo veterinarian or the zoologic facility should consider acquiring if it is routinely used. Quality portable (new or refurbished) microscopes are invaluable for field use for rapid diagnosis using fecal evaluations, skin scrapes, and other cytologies. The veterinarian and/or the facility should have an account with a reference laboratory where samples can be sent for diagnostic testing. If blood samples are collected regularly to be tested off site, a portable centrifuge may be necessary to achieve accurate results. This allows for rapid separation of serum or plasma from cells to ensure more accurate results, and it may also be useful for running on-site packed cell volumes, urine sediments, or centrifuged fecal samples.
- Tuberculosis (TB) testing: intradermal TB testing is an important screening tool to monitor the TB status of a facility's animals and to keep the collection TB-free. For animals that are not readily handleable or approachable, intradermal TB testing is best performed at a site that is readily observed form a distance. Often, the eyelids are used for this purpose. The test should be read by a veterinarian or by qualified personnel at 24, 48, and 72 hours. Although not ideal, if a veterinarian or qualified person is not available to do this, facility personnel can send a veterinarian a digital picture of the test. There are several good references for TB testing in zoologic species.[8–11]

COMMON PROBLEMS AND PROCEDURES

Due to the variety of species of animals that are kept in zoologic collections, there are always new challenges. There are a few situations, however, that tend to be seen and attended to on a regular basis. Although some of these can be scheduled, such as preventative wellness and animal transportation, others may occur on an emergency basis, such as trauma or acute illness.

- Preventative wellness: ideally this should be a scheduled event that allows a veterinarian adequate time to perform all the needed tasks. It may include anesthesia; physical examination; foot, hoof, horn, nail, or dental care; vaccinations and deworming; TB testing; blood, urine, and feces collection for diagnostic testing and sample banking; diagnostic imaging; microchip implantation; reproduction prevention; or any other procedure that is deemed to be necessary based on the species and case.
- Trauma: this includes predator trauma; conspecific aggression; self-trauma (eg, running into a fence); iatrogenic trauma (eg, breaking a leg when recovering from anesthesia); and, in cases of petting zoos and drive-through safaris, injuries caused directly or indirectly by visitors. These incidents can result in wounds and lacerations, fractures, broken horns and antlers, and myriad other injuries, up to and including death. If the injuries are minor, then they may be managed medically via injection, flavored medications, medicated food, or topical medications. If the trauma is serious, then the animal may need to be sedated to address the injury. Severe trauma may necessitate humane euthanasia. Euthanasia techniques should be appropriate for the species.[12,13]
- Field surgery: surgery is best performed in a clean, well-lit, and climate-controlled environment, but there are often situations where this has to be done in less-than-ideal settings. Certainly, trauma often warrants surgical repair of wounds and lacerations, but the author has also performed enucleations, cesarean sections, tumor removals, dental procedures, biopsies, castrations, and many other surgical procedures in a myriad of nonclinical settings.
- Managing infectious diseases: the primary reason that new arrivals are quarantined and sick animals are isolated is to identify potential pathogen transmission before it affects other animals in the collection. Certain infectious diseases can be insidious and difficult to control or prevent. Knowledge of the disease processes that are occurring in a zoologic collection is usually obtained via necropsy/histopathology and laboratory testing. Major morbidity and mortality events may be financially devastating to the zoo. A veterinarian has an obligation to help integrate policies and procedures that reduce both the risk of introduction of new diseases and the transmission of existing pathogens, as well as to monitor these policies and procedures to ensure that they continue to be performed appropriately.
- Veterinary inspections: collections that sell animals or are open to the public are required to have US Department of Agriculture (USDA) permits to operate. One stipulation of this permit is that there has to be a certificate of veterinary inspection that is updated at least annually (discussed previously). The ambulatory zoo veterinarian needs to be familiar with this certification process and be willing and able to hold the zoo accountable for deficiencies.
- Diet and husbandry review: animal husbandry and nutrition are typically the duties of animal keepers, nutritionists, or other similarly trained individuals. It is not uncommon, however, for deficiencies in these areas to lead to animal illness or injury in a zoologic setting. The more knowledgeable veterinarians are about

the captive husbandry of the species within the collection, the more likely they are to be able to identify problem areas, ideally before any animals are injured. New enclosures, diets, enrichment items, landscaping, and species integration into multispecies exhibits should all be scrutinized by the attending veterinarian.

- Theriogenology and neonatology: it is common for zoologic collections to have programs of captive breeding within their collection. An ambulatory veterinarian may be called on to help diagnose reproduction and infertility issues; assess hormone levels; perform semen collection, artificial insemination, or embryo implantation; monitor pregnancy or the incubation of eggs; assist in delivery or hatching; and provide needed veterinary care for the newborns or hatchlings.
- Animal transportation: injuries and death are not uncommon in zoologic species being transported. Often animals must be sedated, anesthetized, or treated with anxiolytic medications to be safely transported. The veterinarian needs to be familiar with these drugs and their effects on an animal being transported, the needs of the animal during transportation, the suitability of the means of transport for the species in question, and proper loading and unloading procedures. In some situations, the veterinarian may be required to travel with the transported animal to provide medical care during the journey. If an animal is transported interstate or internationally, the veterinarian may also be required to provide a health certificate and assist in permit acquisition for that animal prior to shipping (discussed previously).

NECROPSY

As part of preventative medicine in a zoologic setting, necropsies and subsequent pathology and disease testing should be performed on every animal that dies, regardless if the cause of death is known or not. This allows the veterinarian and collection owner to know what pathogenic processes may be present clinically or subclinically within their collection. Necropsies should be performed in a designated area away from other animals and the public to minimize risks associated with the procedure. Smaller collections are often unable to provide this and necropsies are often performed in the field or in multiuse areas. The threat of disease transmission should be taken into consideration for every animal that is undergoing a necropsy. For this reason, personal protection ideally should be worn. Gloves, gowns, masks, and eye protection should be available for this purpose. The instruments used to perform the necropsy (knives, scissors, saws [power and hand], rib cutters, and the like) should be designated for that purpose only. These instruments need to be disinfected or, ideally, sterilized after each use. Specimen containers, formalin, slides, and a variety of sample collection tubes should also be readily available for sample collection.[2,3]

The veterinarian is also ultimately responsible for the final disposition of the animal. Smaller animals can be transported to a veterinary facility or crematorium for disposition. This is often not practical for larger animals. Any animal carcasses that are left at the facility should be either buried or burned or kept in a biologically secure area, such as a deep freezer. Leaving carcasses in the open can result in groundwater contamination or disease transmission via predation, and if the animal was euthanized, scavengers may be poisoned by consuming them. The US Fish and Wildlife Service has determined that if a federally protected species, such as a vulture, is poisoned by the consumption of a euthanized animal that was not properly disposed, the veterinarian who euthanized it as well as the animal's owner are both liable.[14]

Necropsy samples should be submitted to a zoologic pathologist who is knowledgeable about the species submitted and the disease processes that may be of concern. Although this can be a more expensive option, it is also most likely to provide the most usable information. Pathologists who primarily work with domesticated animal specimens can often provide a pathologic diagnosis but may not know what disease processes need to be considered as the etiology. If cost is a factor, a state diagnostic laboratory can be contacted for assistance. In the author's home state (Tennessee), the state diagnostic laboratory runs samples on birds and hoofstock at little or no cost for residents. It should be kept in mind that these state laboratories are often unfamiliar with the species submitted and a pathologic diagnosis may be lacking, but this is a much better option than not submitting samples. The clinician should request the pathology slides be returned or preserved so that they can be sent to a zoologic pathologist if the need arises.

TREATMENT CHALLENGES

Ambulatory zoologic practice is fraught with challenges. When working in the field, veterinarians must deal with the weather, the risk of injury to themselves or to the animals attended to, trauma to conspecifics in the same enclosure, rough terrain or hard-to-access areas, animal transport, prevention of disease transmission, unsanitary environments, and substandard working conditions, to name a few. Cages and enclosures are often not designed with the medical needs of an animal or access by a veterinarian in mind. Many smaller zoos and exotic animal collections often do not have designated keepers for each species of animal kept and may do little or no training or operant conditioning, making diagnosis and treatment difficult and frustrating, particularly for animals with chronic conditions that have to be treated long term. Having a good working relationship with nearby local veterinarians and/or referral centers may be an aid in providing hospitalization or other services that may not be able to be properly performed in the field. Unlike municipal zoos, private zoos, safari parks, and game farms are often operated as for-profit businesses. This means that the bottom line must always be considered, and the owner may choose to euthanize an animal if the cost of veterinary care outweighs the value of the animal. It may also tie the hands of the veterinarian, resulting in the empirical treatment of an animal instead of being able to practice evidence-based medicine. These factors should be discussed with the owners of the collection on the front end, so that the veterinarian knows how far they want to go in a given situation, and clients should also be made aware of the risks associated with doing so. Written documentation of declined veterinary recommendations and signed against medical advice (AMA) forms should ideally be used to limit a veterinarian's liability in these circumstances.

SUMMARY

Ambulatory zoologic veterinary work can be extremely rewarding, but it can also be extremely challenging. Proper preparedness is the key. Being aware of the specific needs of the species being addressed, the working environment, the necessary equipment and supplies, and all the legalities involved leads to more successful outcomes. The successful mobile zoo veterinarian is one who can improvise, adapt, and think outside the box.

REFERENCES

1. Available at: www.aphis.usda.gov/aphis/ourfocus/animalwelfare.
2. Available at: www.aazv.org/resource/resmgr/files/aazvveterinaryguidelines2016. pdf. Accessed December 14, 2017.

3. Miller RE, Fowler ME, editors. Fowler's zoo and wild animal medicine, vol. 8. St Louis (MO): Elsevier; 2015.
4. Kreeger TJ, Arnemo JM. Handbook of wildlife chemical immobilization, 4th edition. Published by author. 2012.
5. West G, Heard D, Caulkett N, editors. Zoo animal and wildlife immobilization and anesthesia. 2nd edition. Ames (IA): Wiley-Blackwell; 2014.
6. Carpenter JW, Marion C, editors. Exotic animal formulary. 5th edition. St Louis (MO): Elsevier; 2018.
7. Available at: www.dea.gov.
8. Lecu A, Ball RL. Recent updates for antemortem tuberculosis diagnostics in zoo animals. In: Miller RE, Fowler ME, editors. Fowler's zoo and wild animal medicine, vol. 8. St Louis (MO): Elsevier; 2015. p. 703–10.
9. Cousins DV, Florrison N. A review of tests available for use in the diagnosis of tuberculosis in non-bovine species. Rev Sci Tech 2005;24(3):1039–59.
10. EAZWV Infectious Disease Working Group. Tuberculosis in zoo species: diagnostic update and management issues. In: transmissible diseases handbook. 4th edition. EAZWV; 2009. Available at: www.eazwv.org/resource/resmgr/Files/Tuberculosis_WG/Infectious_Diseases_Handbook.pdf. Accessed December 14, 2017.
11. Lecu A, Ball RL. Mycobacterial infections in zoo animals: relevance, diagnosis and management. Int Zoo Yb 2011;45:183–202.
12. American Association of Zoo Veterinarians (AAZV). Guidelines for euthanasia of nondomestic animals. 2006. Availbale at: https://www.aazv.org/store/ViewProduct.aspx?id=1905003&hhSearchTerms=%2522euthanasia%2522.
13. Available at: www.avma.org/KB/Policies/Documents/euthanasia.pdf.
14. Leary S, Underwood W, Anthony R, et al. AVMA guidelines for the euthanasia of animals: 2013 edition. Schaumburg (IL): AVMA. Available at: www.in.gov/boah/files/AVMA_Euthanasia_Guidelines.pdf. Accessed December 14, 2017.

Ambulatory Emergency Medicine

James E. Bogan Jr, DVM, DABVP (Canine and Feline Practice),
DABVP (Reptile and Amphibian Practice), CertAqV

KEYWORDS

- Ambulatory • Emergency • Exotic animal • Avian • Reptile

KEY POINTS

- Emergency cases in an ambulatory practice are inevitable.
- Proper emergency preparation is the key to successful case management.
- Equipment and medications required for exotic animal care may be beyond those typically carried for other domestic animal emergencies.
- Being creative and thinking outside of the box are qualities that help the veterinarian through many exotic animal emergency cases in the field.

INTRODUCTION

While practicing exotic animal medicine as an ambulatory practitioner, veterinarians need to be prepared for the inevitable emergency call. Emergencies in exotic animal medicine come in all shapes and sizes and the veterinarian must be prepared for a variety of situations. This article provides a brief overview in managing emergency cases in an ambulatory exotics animal practice.

THE AMBULATORY EXOTIC ANIMAL PRACTITIONER

As an ambulatory exotics veterinarian, the practitioner has the unique advantage to see many species that would be less likely to come into a stationary facility. The client who owns fish, ratites, crocodilians, or venomous reptiles may be better served by a veterinarian who can travel to the patient. Additionally, ambulatory veterinarians may be called to service larger collections (or even small zoologic parks or attractions) because this is more efficient than trying to transport large numbers to a stationary veterinary facility. In these instances, exotic animal emergencies for the ambulatory practitioner may involve a wide array of unique animal species (**Fig. 1**).

Disclosure: The author has nothing to disclose.
The Critter Fixer of Central Florida, PO Box 621679, Oviedo, FL 32762-1679, USA
E-mail address: thecritterfixer@gmail.com

Vet Clin Exot Anim 21 (2018) 699–717
https://doi.org/10.1016/j.cvex.2018.05.006   **vetexotic.theclinics.com**

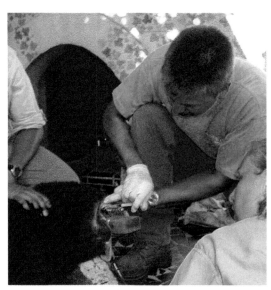

Fig. 1. Local anesthetic being injected before fractured tooth extraction in an anesthetized Florida black bear (*Ursus americanus floridanus*) in the field.

Just as in a traditional stationary veterinary practice, having the proper preparation makes handling emergencies much easier for the ambulatory practitioner. Being prepared means having the proper training, equipment, and medications. In addition, building reliable relationships with stationary veterinary hospitals, referral centers, and emergency clinics can enhance patient care. It is advisable that ambulatory exotic animal veterinarians build a strong rapport with several clinics in their service area. If the ambulatory practitioner can establish "hospital privileges" within any of these veterinary hospitals, emergency cases that need intensive care can be properly managed, enhancing case outcome.

Exotic animal emergencies may not be initially life threatening but need immediate intervention to prevent the situation from escalating into a life-threatening event. A review of basic emergency medicine in exotic animals is essential. The author recommends the review of several references for emergency care in a variety of exotic species.[1–22] It is paramount that the ambulatory practitioner set appropriate expectations for the client and describe the limitations of performing emergency medicine in the field.

EQUIPMENT

Equipment needed in emergency medicine is often the same equipment used for typical exotic animal case management (**Figs. 2–4**). In addition to the typical veterinary equipment, you may need a few items that are unique to emergency medicine. **Box 1** provides a list of potential equipment needs. An important aspect in many emergency situations is the ability to administer oxygen, necessitating the mobile practitioner to carry a portable oxygen delivery system. In most instances, the same portable system that the practitioner may use for anesthesia can double as an emergency oxygen delivery system. Having a variety of anesthetic face masks is needed for the various species seen by the exotic animal practitioner. Clear plastic boxes can be fitted

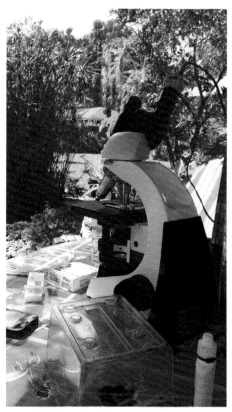

Fig. 2. A portable microscope is an essential piece of equipment in ambulatory medicine. Here a portable microscope is being used to evaluate gill biopsies and skin scrapes as part of a minimum database for an ailing backyard koi (*Cyprinus carpio*).

with oxygen connectors to then be used as oxygen cages, nebulization chambers, or anesthetic induction boxes (**Fig. 5**). Many avian patients with respiratory emergencies may need to be stabilized with oxygen before physical examination. Being creative helps overcome this need in an ambulatory situation. For example, using a clear plastic bag around the bird's cage or carrier with the oxygen hose enclosed is an effective makeshift oxygen tent.

Portable gram scales are important pieces of equipment. Obtaining an accurate weight helps with medication dosage calculations and hydration evaluation. Having clear plastic containers with lockable lids is useful for restraining an animal when obtaining a weight. Make certain that the container has adequate ventilation holes pre-drilled into the sides.

Laryngoscopes and modified otoscopes are useful for visualizing the airway of small patients. Large anesthesia face masks are used as an oxygen chamber for small patients. Having appropriately sized endotracheal tubes for species typically encountered is also a necessity. Often, commercially available endotracheal tubes are too large for many of the smaller patients. Endotracheal tubes can be made out of large intravenous catheters, tomcat catheters, or red rubber feeding tubes. Intubating rabbits and rodents is challenging, especially in an emergency situation.

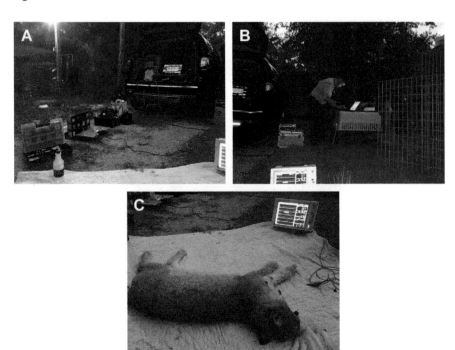

Fig. 3. (*A*) Having a portable blood chemistry machine and digital radiography greatly enhances the diagnostic capabilities for the ambulatory practitioner. Treating larger exotic animals often requires working from your vehicle in the field. (*B*) The ambulatory practitioner working emergencies may need to work outside in low light conditions. Many instances creative use of nearby items is also warranted, such as using a transport crate as make-shift desk. (*C*) Anesthetized Iberian lynx (*Lynx pardinus*). Portable multiparameter monitor being used as a pulse oximeter while animal is on oxygen face mask. The monitor display does not always reveal the pulse oximetry values with consistency, although the monitor produced an audible beep with each heartbeat (note the pulse oximetry waveform on the display). Even when monitoring equipment may be available, do not rely completely on the data presented and always manually double check the patient's physical examination findings.

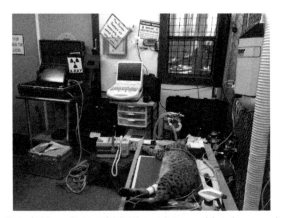

Fig. 4. Portable digital DR radiograph equipment, portable ultrasound equipment, and portable gas anesthesia equipment used on an anesthetized bobcat (*Lynx rufus*). This animal was vomiting after each meal and becoming less active. A gastrotomy was performed on site after diagnosing a gastric foreign body via radiography and ultrasonography.

Box 1
Suggested equipment for exotic animal emergencies

Ambu resuscitation bag

Bandaging material

Cautery (chemical and/or mechanical)

Dart gun/pole syringe

Dissolved oxygen meter

Electrocardiogram unit

Endotracheal tubes

Facemasks

Fiberglass casting tape

Gauze/packing material

Glucometer ± Abaxis iStat

Intravenous catheters

Microscope and slides

Microbial culture tubes and media

Otoscope/laryngoscope

Oxygen tank and regulator

Pulse oximeter

Stethoscope

Surgical adhesive

Suture, absorbable and nonabsorbable

Sterile surgical instrument packs

Syringes and needles

Towels and blankets

Ultrasonography unit

Urinary catheters (various sizes)

Water test kit

Watertight containers

Weight scales

Wood's lamp

The narrow oral opening, elongated soft palate, recessed larynx, small oral cavity, and enlarged tongue can make visualization of the airway difficult. A small rigid or semirigid endoscope with a battery-powered light source can help visualize the airway in rodents. If the clinician is having trouble visualizing the epiglottis in an emergency where obtaining an airway is critical, a tracheostomy can be performed. A tracheostomy should be used as a last resort because of the risk of long-term complications. As an alternative to tracheostomy, inserting a hypodermic needle into the trachea and passing a guidewire through the lumen of the needle and out through the glottis may aid in identifying the airway. Once the guidewire is visible

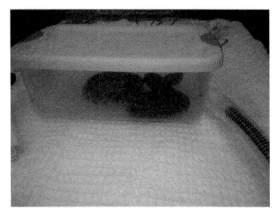

Fig. 5. An eastern diamondback rattlesnake (*Crotalus adamanteus*) in a clear plastic tub fitted to the anesthetic machine.

in the mouth, the veterinarian can then pass an endotracheal tube over the guidewire, through the epiglottis, and into the trachea.

In addition to the emergency-related equipment, there are certain drugs that should also be carried by the ambulatory exotic animal practitioner (**Box 2**). Many of the drugs needed are already in the list of items commonly used, but there are some additional medications that warrant stocking in the ambulatory vehicle. One such example is midazolam. This medication is a benzodiazepine that is water-soluble and is injected intramuscularly or administered intranasally. Multiple studies have shown this drug to be effective in many exotic animal species as a sedative and is used to help them cope with stressful situations.[23–30] Additionally, this drug is easily and safely reversed should a recovery be necessary.

BUSINESS CONSIDERATIONS

Just as with any business, a structured fee schedule is needed to maintain continuity and consistency in an ambulatory practice. An ambulatory veterinary practice should reflect similar fee structures in a traditional stationary facility. It is customary practice to charge an ambulatory fee, or trip charge, for your travel to the location of the animal to be treated. One way to designate charges is to have the ambulatory practice manager map a series of concentric rings around the practice's "home base," reflecting the various levels of ambulatory charges based on distance. As the patient's location becomes farther from the traveling veterinarian's home base, the ambulatory fee increases. Some practices, however, just charge a flat fee for ambulatory travel. This is more appropriate if all clients are located within a similar distance to the traveling veterinarian's home base.

Once on site, there are three main fee structure models typically used to charge for services in the field: (1) traditional, (2) alternative, and (3) contractual. The traditional fee structure is the most common fee structure and it reflects the same structure used in a traditional stationary practice. In this model, the client is charged an ambulatory fee, an examination fee per animal seen, plus appropriate fees for diagnostic tests and treatments completed. The alternative fee structure is often used when large collections are involved. Instead of an examination fee for each animal seen, an hourly rate is charged to the client. This is especially useful for small zoologic collections and breeding facilities that are visited regularly.

Box 2
Suggested medications for exotic animal emergencies

Intravenous fluids (various)

Amphibian ringers

50% dextrose

Appropriate anesthetic agents

Anesthetic reversal agents

Appropriate antimicrobial agents

Aminophylline

Atropine, glycopyrrolate

Calcium gluconate

Dexamethasone

Diphenhydramine

Doxapram

Dopamine

Epinephrine

Furosemide

Heparin

Lidocaine, bupivacaine

Midazolam

MS-222

Physostigmine

Sodium bicarbonate

Syrup of ipecac, apomorphine

Vasopressin

Vitamin K

Vitamin B complex

Vitamin C

Sodium pentobarbital (euthanasia solution)

The contractual fee structure would be used in a situation where the veterinarian has entered into a contract with a business. This business may be a zoologic park, a road-side attraction that displays animals, an aquarium, a science center, or a large breeding operation. Details in the contract vary between facilities but typically involve a monthly stipend to the veterinarian for an agreed number of days per month. This topic is covered in more detail in David Hannon's article, "Ambulatory Zoo Practice," in this issue.

Whichever fee structure is implemented, the fees for emergency situations should be addressed. In a contractual fee structure arrangement, it is best to have fees and expectations spelled out at the time the contract is drafted. In the traditional and alternative fee structures, an emergency fee should be quoted to the client at the time of visit arrangement and added to the invoice at the time of the visit. For

---

Box 3
Common emergencies seen in invertebrates

Chemical intoxication

Trauma

Dysecdysis

Drowning

Hyperthermia

Hypothermia

Constipation

Dehydration

Envenomation

---

example, in the traditional fee structure the client is charged an ambulatory fee, an examination fee, an emergency fee, and fees for diagnostic tests and treatments completed.

Setting expectations for the client at the time the emergency occurs helps the overall case management. Often the ambulatory practitioner must triage cases over the telephone. The use of hands-free devices while driving can allow for a safe continued contact with the distressed client and is the law in most states. The use of video communication (eg, FaceTime or Skype) is also helpful when trying to triage an emergency. Video communication, however, should not be used while driving; the only exception is when the person using the video communication (eg, the veterinarian) is not the person driving the vehicle.

Educating the client in advance of the limitations of what can be done in an ambulatory setting at the time of triage helps with the client's expectations of treatment plan, expected case outcome, and cost of services. During the initial audio or video call, the veterinarian should assess the emergency and determine the appropriate course of action. If the emergency seems to be a situation that may need long-term hospitalization, the veterinarian may instruct the client to meet at one of the stationary clinics where hospital privileges have been established.

Box 4
Common emergencies seen in fish

Ammonia toxicity

Nitrite toxicity

Low dissolved oxygen

Copper toxicity

Pesticide

Gas supersaturation

Buoyancy problems

Infection

Trauma

Box 5
Common emergencies seen in amphibians

Anorexia

Edema

Paresis

Sudden death

Rectal prolapse

Parasites

Sepsis

Gastrointestinal obstruction/foreign body

Bloat

Trauma

Dehydration

Overhydration

COMMON EMERGENCIES

Common emergencies seen in an ambulatory exotic animal practice include true emergencies and perceived emergencies. Perceived emergencies may or may not be true medical conditions but are important for the client and must

---

Box 6
Common emergencies seen in reptiles

Bites

Trauma

Dystocia

Fractures (pathologic vs traumatic)

Gastrointestinal obstruction

Gastrointestinal foreign body

Constipation

Weakness

Hypocalcemia

Retained spectacle

Subspectacular abscess

Prolapse

Renal failure

Drowning

Pneumonia

Thermal burns

Sepsis

Box 7
Common emergencies seen in pet birds

Sinusitis

Tracheal obstruction

Respiratory toxin

Pneumonia

Cardiovascular failure

Crop stasis

Diarrhea/melena

Dystocia

Egg yolk peritonitis

Cloacal prolapse

Seizure

Ataxia and tremors

Head trauma

Acute leg paresis

Broken blood feather

Lacerations

Burns (crop)

Bite wounds

Leg band

String around digit

Glue trap

Fracture

Toxin exposure

---

be respected as an emergency seen in the client's eyes. An example of this is porphyrin staining in rodent's tear film or in rabbit's urine. Thus, it becomes important to respond as appropriate to an emergency, but also to convey clear communication to the client to educate and prevent false emergencies in the future.

Boxes 3–11 provide a basic list of common emergencies seen for particular animal taxonomic groups. One of the more commonly seen emergencies in an ambulatory setting is trauma, common across all taxa. Traumatic injuries are as minor as scratches and scrapes to more severe, such as proptosis, fracture, and death (**Figs. 6–17**).

Unlike emergencies in a stationary veterinary practice, when trauma management is performed in the field an ambulatory setting may provide challenges in maintaining aseptic conditions (**Figs. 18** and **19**). In all cases, minimizing wound contamination from soil and substrate substantially improves successful patient care. The author has found that the extensive use of clean water and saline, clean blankets, tarps, towels, and adhesive disposable drapes greatly improve

Box 8
Common emergencies seen in fowl
Hemorrhage
Trauma
Hypothermic shock
Heat stress
Dyspnea
Lameness
Lead poisoning
Zinc toxicosis
Botulism
Toxins
Diarrhea
Gastrointestinal impaction
Intussusception
Ceolomitis (egg)
Prolapsed oviduct
Dystocia
Phallus prolapse

cleanliness. Wound cultures taken at the time of initial treatment help adjust antibiotic management and improve patient care and outcome.

SUMMARY

Providing complete veterinary care to exotic animals as a mobile practitioner includes managing emergency cases as they arise. Having adequate preparation for an emergency situation is the key for successful case management. With the proper training, equipment, and managing client expectations, an ambulatory exotics animal practitioner can successfully address emergencies.

Box 9
Common emergencies seen in raptors
Trauma
Electrocution
Respiratory disease
Tracheal obstruction
Toxin exposure
Emaciation
Hypoglycemia
Frostbite

Box 10
Common emergencies seen in companion exotic mammals

Vaccine reaction (ferrets)

Hypoglycemia

Adrenal disease (ferrets)

Gastrointestinal foreign body

Cholelithiasis

Congestive heart failure

Chylothorax (ferrets)

Trauma

Anorexia/dysbiosis

Dental disease (rabbits, guinea pigs, chinchillas)

Gastrointestinal stasis

Respiratory disease
  Pasteurella (rabbits)
  Mycoplasma/cilia-associated respiratory bacillus (rats)

Urolithiasis/urinary obstruction

Paraphimosis

Vestibular disease

Fur slip

Dystocia

Heat stroke

Hypothermia

Anorexia/lethargy

Choking

Hypocalcemia

Wobbly hedgehog syndrome (hedgehogs)

Proptosis

Chromodacryorrhea (porphyrin discharge)

Dental disease

Diarrhea and vomiting

Toxin exposure

Box 11
Common emergencies seen in miniature pigs

Shock

Heat stress/heat stroke

Gastroenteritis

Toxin exposure

Salt poisoning

Idiopathic epilepsy

Vomiting and diarrhea

Urinary tract disorders

Sepsis

Dog bite wounds

Dystocia

Trauma

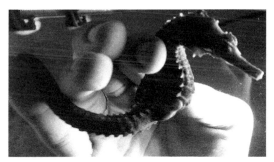

Fig. 6. Spiny sea horse (*Hippocampus histrix*) presented with buoyancy issues. This animal was unable to swim upright and excessive gas was present in the brood pouch. After a diagnosis of gas bubble disease, the animal was successfully treated with aspiration of the gas and injectable ceftazidime and acetazolamide.

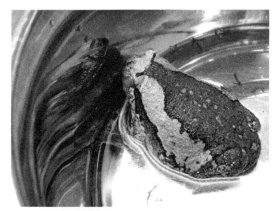

Fig. 7. Asian painted frog (*Kaloula pulchra*) with ruptured globe. Enucleation was performed after tricaine methanesulfate (Finquel MS-222) anesthesia.

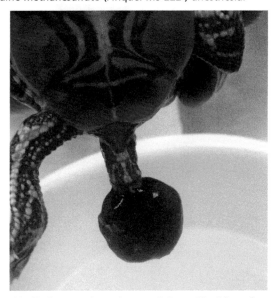

Fig. 8. Northern red-bellied cooter (*Pseudemys rubriventris*) with prolapsed phallus. Cloacal prolapses are not uncommonly seen in chelonian patients and can involve the alimentary, reproductive, and/or urinary tracts. Inspecting the tissue morphology and performing a digital cloacal examination (if possible) and properly identifying the patient's sex can help the practitioner determine which organ has prolapsed.

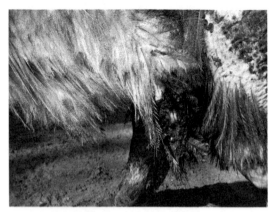

Fig. 9. An emu (*Dromaius novaehollandiae*) with a laceration to the left wing. This bird was injured by a competing male during breeding season.

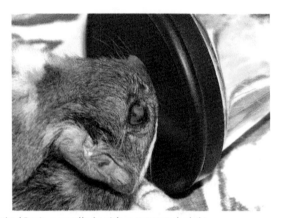

Fig. 10. Guinea pig (*Cavia porcellus*) with a ruptured globe.

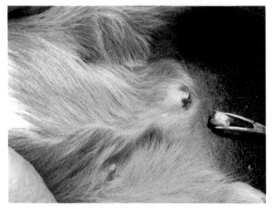

Fig. 11. Male guinea pig (*Cavia porcellus*) with urethral stone. The stone was successfully removed from the anesthetized guinea pig after performing a distal urethrotomy.

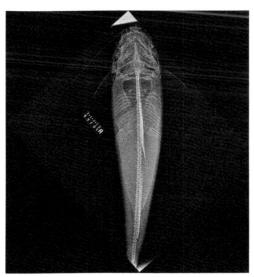

Fig. 12. Dorsoventral radiographic image of a marbled catfish (*Leiarius marmoratus*) with negative buoyancy disorder secondary to trauma. Note the fractures to the third and fourth left ribs.

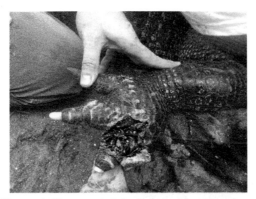

Fig. 13. American alligator (*Alligator mississippiensis*) with a bite wound from another alligator housed in the same pen. Many wounds like this one are managed with minimal intervention in crocodilians. This wound was successfully managed with debridement after local anesthesia and injectable antibiotics. The wound healed well via second intention.

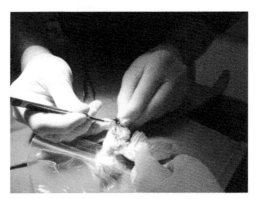

Fig. 14. This zebra finch (*Taeniopygia guttata*) was evaluated for an avulsion trauma involving the right pelvic limb. It was determined that the limb needed to be amputated more proximal for optimal healing. Note the creative use of a zip-lock bag as an anesthesia mask, decreasing the amount of anesthetic gas released into the room.

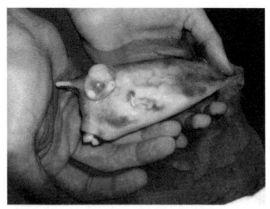

Fig. 15. A longhorn cowfish (*Lactoria cornuta*) with ocular granulomas.

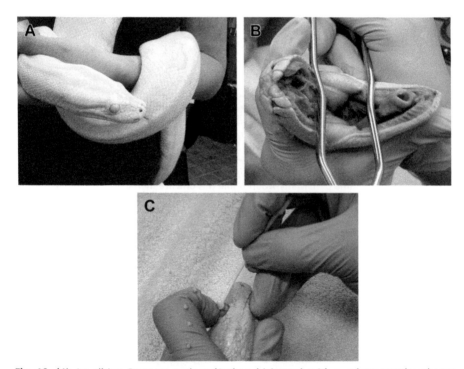

Fig. 16. (*A*) An albino Burmese python (*Python bivittatus*) with a subspectacular abscess involving the right eye. (*B*) A thorough oral examination is required in these cases because many are secondary to infection ascending through the nasolacrimal duct. (*C*) This snake was managed in the field after midazolam sedation and local anesthesia. A pie-shaped wedge was made in the caudoventral portion of the spectacle, a culture obtained, and the caseous material was gently curetted out. Copious lavage succeeded curettage and the patient healed well with antibiotics and husbandry correction.

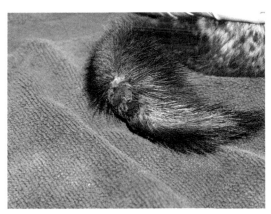

Fig. 17. A chinchilla (*Chinchilla lanigera*) with a tail injury.

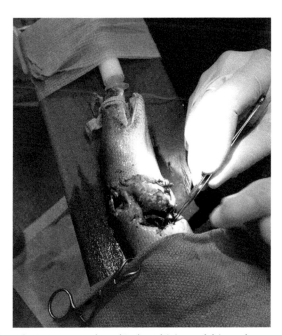

Fig. 18. An adult male Burmese python (*Python bivittatus*) bitten by an adult male reticulated python (*Python reticulatus*). The bite shredded the skin and underlying muscle and lacerated the esophagus and transected the right jugular vein and trachea. The ambulatory setting was a less than ideal surgical location but because of the extensive nature of the wounds, surgery had to be performed on site. A composite deck board placed on sawhorses was used as a surgical table. The surgical site was treated as a clean-contaminated field. Once the snake was anesthetized, the trachea was anastomosed, the esophageal rent closed, the jugular vein ligated, and the muscles and skin were opposed as best as possible. The animal was placed on antibiotics for 4 weeks and the wound healed without incident.

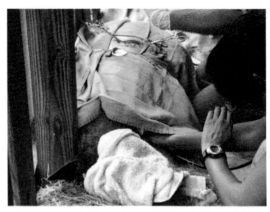

Fig. 19. Emergency rumenotomy in the field on an anesthetized fallow deer (*Dama dama*). This animal ingested a plastic bag. This procedure was completed with injectable anesthetics and local nerve blocks.

REFERENCES

1. Costello MF. Principles of cardiopulmonary cerebral resuscitation in special species. Sem Avian Exot Pet Med 2004;13:132–41.
2. Lichtenberger M, Richardson JA. Emergency care and managing toxicoses in the exotic animal patient. Vet Clin North Am Exot Anim Pract 2008;11:211–28.
3. Cooper JE. Emergency care of invertebrates. Vet Clin North Am Exot Anim Pract 1998;1:251–64.
4. Dombrowski D, De Voe R. Emergency care of invertebrates. Vet Clin North Am Exot Anim Pract 2007;10:621–45.
5. Marnell C. Tarantula and hermit crab emergency care. Vet Clin North Am Exot Anim Pract 2016;19:627–46.
6. Lewbart GA. Emergency and critical care of fish. Vet Clin North Am Exot Anim Pract 1998;1:233–49.
7. Hadfield CA, Whitaker BR, Clayton LA. Emergency and critical care of fish. Vet Clin North Am Exot Anim Pract 2007;10:647–75.
8. Crawshaw GJ. Amphibian emergency and critical care. Vet Clin North Am Exot Anim Pract 1998;1:207–31.
9. Clayton LA, Gore SR. Amphibian emergency medicine. Vet Clin North Am Exot Anim Pract 2007;10:587–620.
10. Martinez-Jimenez D, Hernandez-Divers SJ. Emergency care of reptiles. Vet Clin North Am Exot Anim Pract 2007;10:557–85.
11. Music MK, Strunk A. Reptile critical care and common emergencies. Vet Clin North Am Exot Anim Pract 2016;19:591–612.
12. Stout JD. Common emergencies in pet birds. Vet Clin North Am Exot Anim Pract 2016;19:513–41.
13. González MS, Carrasco DC. Emergencies and critical care of commonly kept fowl. Vet Clin North Am Exot Anim Pract 2016;19:543–65.
14. Graham JE, Heatley JJ. Emergency care of raptors. Vet Clin North Am Exot Anim Pract 2007;10:395–418.
15. Hawkins MG, Graham JE. Emergency and critical care of rodents. Vet Clin North Am Exot Anim Pract 2007;10:501–31.

16. Schnellbacher R, Olson EE, Mayer J. Emergency presentations associated with cardiovascular disease in exotic herbivores. J Exot Pet Med 2012;21:316–27.

17. DeCubellis J. Common emergencies in rabbits, guinea pigs, and chinchillas. Vet Clin North Am Exot Anim Pract 2016;19:411–29.

18. Pollock C. Emergency medicine of the ferret. Vet Clin North Am Exot Anim Pract 2007;10:463–500.

19. Di Girolamo N, Selleri P. Medical and surgical emergencies in ferrets. Vet Clin North Am Exot Anim Pract 2016;19:431–64.

20. McLaughlin A, Strunk A. Common emergencies in small rodents, hedgehogs, and sugar gliders. Vet Clin North Am Exot Anim Pract 2016;19:465–99.

21. Riley J, Barron H. Wildlife emergency and critical care. Vet Clin North Am Exot Anim Pract 2016;19:613–26.

22. Tynes VV. Emergency care for potbellied pigs. Vet Clin North Am Exot Anim Pract 1998;1:177–89.

23. Mans C, Guzman DS, Lahner LL, et al. Sedation and physiologic response to manual restraint after intranasal administration of midazolam in Hispaniolan Amazon parrots (Amazona ventralis). J Avian Med Surg 2012;26:130–9.

24. Sadegh AB. Comparison of intranasal administration of xylazine, diazepam, and midazolam in budgerigars (Melopsittacus undulatus): clinical evaluation. J Zoo Wildl Med 2013;44:241–4.

25. Schroeder CA, Smith LJ. Respiratory rates and arterial blood gas tensions in healthy rabbits given buprenorphine, butorphanol, midazolam, or their combinations. J Am Assoc Lab Anim Sci 2011;50:205–11.

26. Cortright KA, Wetzlich SE, Craigmill AL. Plasma pharmacokinetics of midazolam in chickens, turkeys, pheasants and bobwhite quail. J Vet Pharmacol Ther 2007;30:429–36.

27. Kubiak M, Roach L, Eatwell K. The influence of a combined butorphanol and midazolam premedication on anesthesia in psittacid species. J Avian Med Surg 2016;30:317–23.

28. Santangelo B, Micieli F, Mozzillo T, et al. Transnasal administration of a combination of dexmedetomidine, midazolam and butorphanol produces deep sedation in New Zealand White rabbits. Vet Anaesth Analg 2016;43:209–14.

29. Oppenheim YC, Moon PF. Sedative effects of midazolam in red-eared slider turtles (Trachemys scripta elegans). J Zoo Wildl Med 1995;26:409–13.

30. Arnett-Chinn ER, Hadfield CA, Clayton LA. Review of intramuscular midazolam for sedation in reptiles at the National Aquarium, Baltimore. J Herp Med Surg 2016;26:59–63.

Moving?

Make sure your subscription moves with you!

To notify us of your new address, find your **Clinics Account Number** (located on your mailing label above your name), and contact customer service at:

Email: journalscustomerservice-usa@elsevier.com

800-654-2452 (subscribers in the U.S. & Canada)
314-447-8871 (subscribers outside of the U.S. & Canada)

Fax number: 314-447-8029

Elsevier Health Sciences Division
Subscription Customer Service
3251 Riverport Lane
Maryland Heights, MO 63043

*To ensure uninterrupted delivery of your subscription, please notify us at least 4 weeks in advance of move.